PRAISE FOR THE TRA.
POWER OF SOUND AND MUSIC:

"Out of the many books written about the healing aspects of music, *The Transformational Power of Sound and Music* by Flicka Rahn and Tammy McCrary rises to the top. This handbook explains how and why music allows us to experience our Divine selves. As we move into this emerging era of unity, one of the most powerful ways to connect one heart to another is through music. This is the guide to give you practical keys for this unity connection, using music for profound spiritual transformation."

—**Michael Bernard Beckwith,** founder and spiritual director, Agape International Spiritual Center

"It is rare to find a music industry executive who shares such practical yet heartfelt knowledge about the power and influence that music has on the listener's body, mind, and spirit, In her chapter, 'The Emerging Vision of Sound Healing in the Twenty-First Century,' Tammy McCrary shines the light on the importance of musicians taking a conscious and responsible approach to music making."

—**Marianne Williamson**

"Flicka and Tammy have masterfully written THE HANDBOOK for artists to consciously take their music to the next level. *The Transformational Power of Sound and Music* is a must-read for all music makers."

—**Chaka Khan,** Grammy Award-winning recording artist

"One of the most powerful things about Flicka Rahn is that she knows the field of music from top to bottom and inside out. She is a student, a teacher, a renowned performer, and a shaman. Add to that her depth study of the quantum field, plus her own personal journey of going out to the edges of the newest scientific studies of energy, emotion, and vibration, and you arrive at a brand-new, exciting present moment, ushering in a new version of the early beginnings of the Aquarian Age. Flicka Rahn's new ideas offer healing of mind and body in depth, "stretching" of beliefs and thoughts, thereby birthing new feelings and behaviors. I found every chapter to be engaging, interesting, and inspirational—as well as enlightening."

—**Marjorie R. Barlow, Ph.D.,** consultant, positive psychology, mentoring, and relationships, and author of *The Possible Woman*

"Flicka Rahn's book comes to us in the midst of a revolution of health and healing. She brilliantly brings together the ancient history of music of sound that provides the foundation for our understanding of how greatly powerful sound and music can be in health and wellness. She eloquently tells of ancient traditions of using certain rhythms, sounds, and vibration and then delves into the scientific research that supports sound and music as a way to deeply heal the human mind body spirit and soul. Sound helps to facilitate shifts in our brainwave state by using what we now call *entrainment*. Entrainment synchronizes our fluctuating brainwaves by providing a stable frequency which the brainwave can attune to and by using rhythm and frequency. This can be not only relaxing in our stress-filled world but massively therapeutic. It is no wonder that this ancient tradition of sound and music is making a modern-day renaissance—we have never needed it more!"

—**Suzanne K. Gazda, M.D.**, neurologist and humanitarian, founder, Destiny Health and Wellness and HopeforHumans.org

"*The Transformational Power of Sound and Music* is a groundbreaking book, filled with enlightening teachings on the use of sound, music, intention, ritual, and ultimately, the energy of Love as healing modalities. The book combines ancient wisdom, indigenous spiritual practices, and the latest scientific research in subtle energy to deliver a comprehensive healing manual that should be read by all healers and musicians. Eloquently written and thought provoking."

—**João Mendes and Ramiro Mendes,** musicians, humanitarians, and authors of *Sound: The Fabric of Soul, Consciousness, Reality, and the Cosmos*

"As an experienced healer following the Amazonian Shipibo healing traditions, I found that Flicka Rahn and Tammy McCrary's book, *The Transformational Power of Sound and Music,* is an invaluable guide for all healers. Rich and deep shamanic wisdom is revealed to the reader as Rahn describes her experience with the songs (*icaros*) and sounds present in the ayahuasca ceremonies. She describes the physical and psychological effect of specific sounds and songs and how they can heal the spirit. Having spent years with the Shipibo Indians, I can attest that her discoveries are valid. Her music echoes the profound healing domain just beyond our awareness. Techniques and practical tools using sound as a sonic bridge to wholeness and peace are also described in this book. Rahn and McCrary always return the reader to the only true reality, which is the energy of compassion and love."

—**Yunuen Ramirez,** shaman of ayahuasca and Mexican alternative therapies

"WOW! *The Transformational Power of Sound and Music* by Flicka Rahn and Tammy McCrary is a game changer. Anyone in the movement of unity consciousness, spiritual ascension, spiritual and sound healing, and conscious evolution needs this book. I loved it! Both Flicka and Tammy share deep knowledge of music and sound by telling their personal stories. The book reads like an adventure novel."

—**Alanna Luna,** owner of Newman Media, director and producer of *Sonic Geometry*

"As a psychologist, my aim is to help clients create harmonious lives. It impresses me that sound and music can be a pathway to calming our emotions and restoring inner peace. Rahn and McCrary have done brilliant work in this book explaining how we may empower ourselves to heal and soothe body, mind, and soul, an essential capability in the stressful world in which we live."

—**Davina Kotulski, Ph.D.,** psychologist and author of
It's Never Too Late to be Your Self

"Every shaman should read this book. Shamans attune with the unseen, elemental forces of nature that surround and move through us by entering nonordinary states of consciousness. In this handbook for musicians and sound healers, Rahn and McCrary reveal how and why certain musical tones and percussive rhythms have such a powerful impact on our brains and bodies--down to the cellular level—so we may utilize them to shift our consciousness and heal."

—**Renee Baribeau,** shaman, soul coach, and author of
Winds of Spirit: Ancient Wisdom Tools for Navigating Relationships, Health, and the Divine

"Music is one of the most powerful tools available for creating sacred space and harmony in our homes, workplaces, and environments. It has the sublime power to transform mood, feelings, and ambiance; whether to uplift and energize or to soothe and comfort. Plus, it gives us the ability to tap into the entire spectrum of emotions regulating our wellbeing. As a longtime meditation practitioner with a passion for the soulful art of feng shui and with a master's degree in Consciousness Studies, I wholeheartedly endorse *The Power of Transformational Music and Sound.* Read it and then experiment with the techniques the authors recommend. You'll be amazed with its power of transformation!"

—**Shawne Mitchell, M.A.,** author of
Home Sanctuaries and *Exploring Feng Shui*

"As a professional musician with a lifelong interest and dedication in linking music and sound as a healing path, I wholeheartedly recommend *The Transformational Power of Sound and Music* by Flicka Rahn and Tammy McCrary. To my delight, their expansive study ranges from the earliest roots of shamanic healing on up through twenty-first-century pioneers in this exciting field. With the authors' deft approach in grounding once considered esoteric experience with solid scientific research of our day, this important information has the power to reach and inspire a wide audience. A profound call to resonate to a divine frequency."

—**Wendy Luck, Ph.D.,** flutist, vocalist, composer, multi-media/recording artist, and sound healer. Her solo flute CD, *The Ancient Key,* was recorded inside the King's Chamber in the Great Pyramid of Egypt. Author of *The Therapeutic and Healing Effects of Music and Sound* and *Flute, Voice, Muse, and Multimedia: Creating a Work of Performance Art*

"For fifteen years, I officed down the hallway from Flicka Rahn. Her wisdom as a musical healer, grounded in an incredible musical talent and extensive scientific research, provided insight and tools that allowed me to excel in the face of new challenges and pressures. Through this book others can now share in those priceless gifts."

—**Kelly Quintanilla, Ph.D.,** professor of communications

THE TRANSFORMATIONAL POWER OF SOUND AND MUSIC

···

A HANDBOOK FOR SOUND HEALERS AND MUSICIANS

FLICKA RAHN, M.M.ED., M.SC.
AND TAMMY MCCRARY

Life in 432 Publishing
BEVERLY HILLS, CALIFORNIA

Life in 432 Publishing
www.lifein432.com

Cover design by Alanna Newman, Newman Media
Copy editing and book production by Stephanie Gunning
Book Layout © 2018 Book Design Templates

Ordering Information:
Quantity sales. Special discounts are available on quantity purchases by corporations, associations, and others. For details, contact the publishers at the website above.

Library of Congress Control Number: 2018913102

The Transformational Power of Sound and Music/Flicka Rahn and Tammy McCrary. —1st ed.
ISBN 978-1-7328599-0-6

CONTENTS

*This book is dedicated to the memory of
Henry and Evelyn Rahn, whose love
and support are eternal*

....

HOW AND WHY I BECAME
A SOUND HEALER

I've always been in love with music. This love affair began in the womb. My mother was a classical violinist, so the earliest sounds I heard were her voice and the exquisitely beautiful sounds of her violin. As an infant, I can recall sitting in my crib listening to Bach, Schubert, and Mendelssohn string quartets. Mom and Dad played in a string quartet together and rehearsals for their concerts were held at our home.

Our living room had a piano. When I was old enough to reach the keyboard, I would delicately test the notes, gradually learning to run my fingers up and down the scale as if I was learning a language—or perhaps remembering a language I had known intimately in another lifetime. I sang constantly and would ask any visitors to our home if I could sing for them. They always said yes. In this way, a professional singer was molded from the age of four. I can remember, even from that early age, that music and singing had the power to return me to a place in myself that was known and cherished.

Music was sonic comfort for me. I used music to express myself—making up little songs about my life experiences. My mother, the family's best-trained musician, put my songs into written music for me. I have that special sheet music still; my favorite composition is "Little Dead Bird," which I sang after a sad discovery of a fallen sparrow. I was about six when that song was composed.

When I was eight, I had a profound experience that opened the way for me to experience music as a transcendental medium. It was a beautiful Texas afternoon and I was lying on my back in the front yard, watching clouds moving gently across the sky. As I lay there, mind wandering, I experienced a burst of clarity and awareness, much like the feeling I got when I was singing. I knew I was somehow connected to the clouds above me. And I was in awe at the mystery of the feeling of unity, which was more familiar and powerful than any sensation I had ever consciously experienced.

This memory is emblazoned on my heart: To this day, I can remember the smell of the grass, the sensation of the warmth on my back from the earth, and the gentleness of the breeze as it moved over my face. Certainly, as a young child I could not fully understand what was happening. Looking back, I realize I had briefly connected with the Divine

Presence and received my first tiny glimpse of expanded awareness.

As I matured, whenever I immersed myself in music, either listening or performing, I experienced a similarly expanded state of awareness.

My Musical Training

My life's journey guided me further into the world of music. My family moved to Pittsburgh, Pennsylvania, where I was enrolled in Mount Lebanon High School. I was a member of the school chorus and also sang in the choir at the local Methodist church. I took piano and voice lessons as a teenager and continued to build my skills as a musician. During the last two years of high school, I secured a delightful job as a soloist singing for the Christian Science Church on Sundays. I had to learn a new solo every week, which I would practice with the organist right before the service. This was a great way to sharpen my music reading skills and I loved it. I was also an enthusiastic member of the Mount Lebanon High School Triple Trio, a woman's vocal group of nine singers. We traveled around Pittsburgh and performed for many civic groups, hospitals, and nursing homes. My church and school solidly supported my education as a performer.

After graduating from high school, I attended Washington University in St. Louis, Missouri, as a music major. I could not envision another path of study for myself except music and my parents were 100 percent behind my decision. However, they did encourage me to get a degree in music education rather than music performance, as they wanted me to ensure I could support myself after college. This was excellent advice.

Loving choral music as I did, I joined the Washington University Madrigal Singers. This helped me to cultivate in-depth knowledge of musical style and eloquence. Through my coursework, I began to appreciate the subtleties and majesty of classical music. I studied the great musical masters and found that there was a world of unimaginable beauty in their music. The sublime world of Bach's music and the heart-wrenchingly beautiful music of Fauré and Puccini are perhaps my favorites. My discerning ear was emerging. Soon I could differentiate every musical line played by any instrument within the massive sonic wall of an orchestral performance.

After earning a bachelor's degree in music education, I took a job teaching elementary music in the Pittsburgh School District. I was what was cheerfully called a member of the *traveling faculty*. As an itinerant music teacher, I traveled to four schools and saw every child in the district once a week. Each class was about thirty minutes long, and the pace was massively exhausting, but I had a job to do and I did it. My skills at handling large groups of people were called to task, especially when those people were children in grade school.

In the midst of all this, I got married and gave birth to a precious little girl who continues to be the light of my life today as an adult. Life continued to call me to expand my experience when she was an infant. My next job was in San Antonio, Texas, as a music teacher in (thankfully) ONE school. I can remember showing my class a video of *Amahl and the Night Visitors* by Gian Carlo Menotti. Composed and broadcast on television in 1951, it is a delightful opera. As I viewed the opera with my students, I had the clear realization that I wanted to go back to school and earn a master's degree in vocal performance. Catalyzed by my deep love for singing, I enrolled at Texas State University in San Marcos, Texas. There, I realized that my talent as an operatic soprano was substantial.

While at Texas State, I sang in the University's productions of *Carmen* (as Carmen) and *La Bohème* (as Mimi). I composed countless songs: choral pieces for churches and temples, children's songs, and instrumental pieces for piano. Music was part of every breath I took. It filled my lungs and defined my life.

Along with the comprehensive knowledge I was acquiring of music theory, history, and composition, vocal technique and literature, and piano performance, I was aware of the deepening of another kind of knowledge—knowledge of the magic and mystery of sound. That awareness was never "learned," it was a deep knowing that came as natural to me as breathing. I understood innately that music has the power to evolve the soul, as I felt it consistently urging me toward a fuller expression of my true self.

Music was the sacred land, the temple of peace, the healing stone I would go to daily. Whenever I would perform and sing, I did so from a state of expanded awareness. Time would stand still as I became unaware of myself and yet remained deeply connected to my audience, in a profound experience of unity. The seeds of a sound healer were beginning to grow in me.

My Early Career

After graduation, I was hired by Incarnate Word College in San Antonio, Texas, as a vocal professor. Along with faculty recitals and college opera productions, I sang with the San Antonio Opera Company and began to get real professional experience as an opera singer. This was also the time that I composed many art songs, which are poems set to music and sung by one voice accompanied by a piano. A few of these songs would later be published in the sheet music compilation *Art Songs by American Women Composers, Volume 10* (Southern Music Company, 1995). I traveled across the United States and Asia with my dear friend Ruth Friedberg as my accompanist, performing my songs as well as others by American women.

In 1978, my husband and I and our nine-year-old daughter moved to Boston, Massachusetts. My husband was a brilliant surgeon and eager to be a part of the medical community on the East Coast, and I was similarly eager to be part of the music scene. However, the marriage soon ended, and I was faced with supporting my daughter and myself. I found a job teaching voice in the Graduate Theater Program at Brandeis University. This commenced a ten-year period of incredible productivity for me. I quickly found a home at the Boston Lyric Opera Company. I also sang for opera companies from Minneapolis to New York and sang many oratorios and concert pieces with symphony orchestras. A highlight during this period was performing the soprano solos in Mahler's Second Symphony with the Boston Philharmonic Symphony at Carnegie Hall. My career as an opera singer was proceeding beautifully, as was my career as a music instructor.

As you can see, life was rich and challenging and my career was exciting. And it was going to get even more exciting when my relationship to sound and music went in a new direction.

A Brush with Enlightenment

Music instigated a second brush with enlightenment that was much like the experience I had as a child merging with the clouds. This event took place on the Connecticut Turnpike as I was returning from my uncle's funeral in Philadelphia. I was listening to Pachelbel's Canon, truly one of the most beautiful and moving orchestral pieces I know. Alone in my car, tears streaming down my face as I mourned my uncle's passing, my heart was wide open. Suddenly, without warning, I was enveloped in a tube of brilliant white light. The love that I felt flooding into my heart in that moment surpassed any I had ever before experienced. Nearly blinded by tears, I pulled my car off the Turnpike. If I could have, I would have stayed in that expanded state for eternity. I would have gladly left my life as I knew it behind, to stay suspended there in that bliss.

There on the shoulder of the road, I remained enveloped in light for at least a couple of minutes, though I honestly don't really know how long it lasted as time felt like both an eternity and a split second. As I slowly returned to my earthly awareness, I realized that I had been forever changed. I knew then that I was part of that light—one with it—just as I had known as a little girl that I was connected to the clouds. I had found this light with an open heart and on the wings of beautiful music.

I share this experience with you, as it seemed to set the stage for many subsequent transcendental experiences. A pattern was forming with music and expanded consciousness. Except for the childhood experience, music was always involved in altering my awareness.

Life Changes, Leading to a
New Direction

In 1988, I began to feel that my time in Boston was drawing to an end. My daughter was off to college and the rent on my little house in Boston was rising by the second. I can't say that I was looking for a husband, but during a trip to Corpus Christi, Texas, to sing with the Corpus Christi Opera I met the man who was to become my second husband. Later that year, as a new wife, I moved to Corpus Christi to begin my new life. I was coming home to the city where I was born and where my parents still lived. After arriving, I secured a job as a tenure track member of the music faculty at Texas A&M University, teaching studio voice. This was a period of conflicting feelings for me. My marriage as a peaceful partnership was not working whereas my teaching at the university was expanding toward exciting new horizons. The stress I was experiencing as a result of discord in my marriage was unbearable and my teaching at the university was suffering. My second husband and I divorced after a year of marriage.

Because my personal life and marital choices had proven to be so painful, I entered psychotherapy to figure out why I had chosen such a difficult a path for myself. My psychotherapist happened also to be a faculty member in the guidance and counseling program at the university where I taught. She recognized in me the insatiable drive to understand the human condition and encouraged me to become a trained counselor myself. I knew from personal experience that music and sound are great resources for coping with physical, emotional, and spiritual crises. I could see how music would be of tremendous assistance in returning people to a state of mental health and wellbeing and agreed that expanding my abilities would enable me to be a healer and guide. I had experienced the sanctuary of a safe harbor within myself with music. Sometimes during the preceding painful year, it was the only safe harbor I had.

Two years later, I was awarded a master's degree in guidance and counseling from Texas A&M University, Kingsville. The formal education I received was invaluable as a way of understanding the way the human mind works and creates its own reality. I began to see and experience the psychological benefit of music, sound, and singing. I brought all of this knowledge to my university students as I helped them to explore their inner struggles. To that end, I created two university courses which were related to the transformational power of sound. These were "The Healing Nature of Music and Sound," which I taught with my music faculty colleague Arlene Long, and "Self-Esteem Through Singing and Speaking." Both courses were extremely popular with the students of all disciplines. From the School of Nursing to the School of Business, this knowledge was universally desired and valued.

As voice teacher, I had become a way-shower for my students. Having long seen myself as a servant to my art—whether I was teaching, performing, directing, or composing—using music as a modality for physical, emotional, and spiritual healing was a natural next step.

Eventually, my personal insights begged the question "Could music and sound do the same for others as it has done for me?" I knew that music had the power to remind me of who I truly am. Also, I knew that music had the power to move me past the limitations of my beliefs, conditioning, ego, and judgment.

Feeling as though I was now on a quest, I began looking for universal elements in sacred, spiritual, and meditative music from all over the world, from which I hoped to discern principles of healing with sound and voice. The Tama-Do Academy of Sound, Color, and Movement, based in Malibu, California, offered summer courses in France and I registered to attend. This was my formal introduction to the mystical world of sound—both experienced and studied. Fabian Maman is the director of this school that offers training in the application of tuning forks to acupuncture points, the effects of colored light in healing, and qigong movement therapy. From him I learned that blockages in our subtle energy fields can result in physical illnesses if they are allowed to persist, and that sound is an incredibly effective tool for dissolving these blocks. I am such an admirer of Maman, who was the first researcher to experiment rigorously, under laboratory conditions, with sound and cellular biology. His course set me on a clear path in my own research. Having recognized that sound, music, science, and gathering objective data were clearly the way of the future, it was important for me to study music from this perspective— as well as to acknowledge and exhibit what I instinctively knew worked.

After twenty-three years at Texas A&M, my tenure as an academic drew to an end. Massive life changes were clearly on the horizon as I had also recently remarried for the third time. This was a marriage of quiet peace and total mutual support. I finally found my life partner and best friend. After deep consideration, my husband and I decided to move from Corpus Christi to north of San Antonio, Texas, to fulfill our dream of living in the beautiful Texas Hill County. There we could enjoy the peace of the rolling hills and could stable and pasture my beloved horses. Our arrival on the land was a pause in my life that gave me the opportunity to get in touch with my deepest desire: to be of service through the mystical medium of sound and music. I wanted to formalize this service by becoming a sound therapist. Opening an office at the Integrative Healing Institute in downtown San Antonio, I began to put the breadth of my knowledge of music to work.

Soon after our move to the Hill Country, I took a trip to Mexico to visit friends and had the opportunity to be a part of a sacred plant ceremony facilitated by shaman Yunuen Ramirez. My worldview changed that night. Suddenly I saw multiple dimensions in my physical reality, full of magnificent light, color, and sound, overlaid on one another. What I had "known" in my heart intuitively was displayed before me as a reality that is as concrete as the one we live in. Every shape has a sound, and our bodies are humming with soundwaves. I saw that the world is an interactive web of sound and light that we can consciously affect with our intentions. There are sacred sounds embedded everywhere that hold the keys to perpetual harmony. I knew that I was to offer this deeper knowing to others in many ways: as a sound healer, a sound therapist, a composer, a teacher of the deeper mysteries, and as a performer.

Recording an album of meditation music was my first goal. I asked my dear friend and accompanist, Daniel Wyman, if he would venture into a new world with me and create this project of mystical sound built on the resonant pitches of eight major chakras in the human body, and he enthusiastically agreed. I knew the elements of music and sound I wanted to incorporate and utilize to create a healing landscape.

The actual recording of the tracks took only one and a half days, as all the music was improvised. Nothing was written down or notated prior to the recording. We trusted in the flow of sound coming through to guide us, and it did. We did not repeat or redo any of the eight tracks on that album. Daniel and I both went into a semi-trance state as the sound flowed forth from our voices and instruments, time stood still, and something greater and deeper was in charge. We entitled the album *Icaros: Chakra Soundscapes* in honor of the Shipibo healers of the Peruvian Amazon who often will sing their medicine. We intended for our songs to be sacred songs, *icaros*, that would enable westerners to connect with the divine space within themselves.

This deeper knowledge and view into the metaphysical effects and elements of sound and music has defined my path since that night in Mexico. With this book, I offer you the fruits of my years of research and the discoveries and personal observations I have made into the mystery of music. Insights continue to emerge. We are at an exciting intersection where sound and frequency are becoming widely accepted and recognized healing modalities. I am grateful to the many brilliant philosophers, musicians, and scientists whose knowledge and research have elucidated my direct experience of the power of transformational and healing music.

As you journey through this book, you will be introduced to the principles of healing with sound and music, both instrumental and vocal, and learn how and why it is effective. We will cover the many roots of ancient and indigenous healing music, which extend from ancient Egypt and Medieval Europe to the present day, and discover the seeds of healing within the sonic traditions of diverse cultures. Having reviewed that vast expanse of information, we will then begin to look at the specific sounds, keys, intervals, and instruments that are common elements in different healing traditions and explore the reasons why. Having delved into that body of knowledge, like a sonic surgeon, we will discuss the effects of frequency and sound on our psychological states, physical bodies, and subtle energy. To put this knowledge to practical use, we will learn how to use the many options for sound healing to heal ourselves and others.

To conclude our journey, the last chapter of this book, written by artist manager Tammy McCrary, will describe a visionary map of the future of sound in healing the twenty-first century.

....

ONE

A WORLD HISTORY OF SPIRITUAL MUSIC THAT HEALS

Worldwide, there is a robust history of healing music. To understand the current movement of spiritual awakening through music, sound, and meditation we must understand and explore the music of our ancestors. This ancient knowledge is the wellspring of the emerging horizon in sound therapy today.

Indigenous Peoples, Ancient Healing Traditions, and Sound

The ancient world was rich with healing modalities. Music—and sound in general—was deeply valued by native shamans, priests, and priestesses and early physicians. Sound therapy was widely known and practiced as an effective method of returning a diseased body and spirit to a state of health and wholeness. As you read about these traditions you may recognize many similarities to present day practices with sound healing. To fully understand the power of sound, I needed to dig deep into the ancestral roots of the healers that have gone before me. I felt that there were gems of knowledge awaiting me and I was not wrong. Read the following like a sonic detective on the quest for truth. The ultimate questions I asked were: Why did the ancients use those specific sounds to heal? What was it about those sounds? Why did those sounds work?

Ancient Egypt

Our earliest reports of sound healing—specifically sung vowel sounds—date back to the Egyptian culture around 4000 B.C.E. It was reported by Demetrius, a Greek visiting Egypt around 200 B.C.E., that Egyptians used vowel sounds in their ceremonies. "In Egypt, when priests sing hymns to the gods, they sing the seven vowels in due succession and the sound has such euphony that men listen to it instead of the flute and the lyre"[1]

The *Corpus Hermeticum* offers a reference to the use of sound in spiritual awareness. These Egyptian wisdom texts, originally thought to be from the first century C.E., probably date further back, perhaps even to 1400 B.C.E. The texts are written as lessons to be given to a disciple. Further reference to vowels used in ceremony is taken from writing attributed to Asclepius-Imhotep, circa 2500 B.C.E., in which he says, "As for us, we do not use simple words but sounds all filled with power."[2] These references to vowel sounds as possessing healing properties made perfect sense to me as any vocalist worth his or her salt knows that vowels carry energy, intention, and vitality.

Not only were vocal sounds used in antiquity for healing; percussion instruments were as well.

It is interesting to note that one of the instruments used in ceremony in ancient Egypt was a sistrum, a rattle with metal disks strung on lines suspended between two wooden poles. In reflecting on the sound of the sistrum, we know that it is very rich in ultrasound, which lies above 40,000 hertz (Hz). Our modern-day cymbal produces ultrasound up into the 100,000 Hz range. Ultrasound technology is used today by physical therapists to stimulate muscle repair and relieve joint discomfort. This very-high-frequency sound is way above our ability to hear it, as normal hearing ranges from 20–20,000 Hz. And, as we age, we do not hear the upper frequencies. So, it is entirely possible that percussive sound of the sistrum enhanced and expanded the soundscape of the ceremonies, and also was used to enhance healing by creating an ultrasonic fabric. That sound would have been greatly enhanced within a resonant chamber.

For both secular and religious occasions, stringed instruments, such as harps and lyres, were used in small ensembles, as well as flutes and oboes. Interestingly, a pentatonic scale—a musical scale with five notes instead of the seven common in western music—was used as a basis for compositions and performances, which were all improvised. What we know about pentatonic scales is that any two notes from the scale can be sounded together without dissonance. This means the sound from the harps, flutes, and percussion instruments common in Egyptian ceremonies would have blended together beautifully. Clapping was another form of percussion always present in the ensembles. There were singers too.

Ancient Egyptian physicians describe specific musical songs for healing the sick. Many contemporary researchers, notably John Stuart Reid, have done extensive research on the healing sound created within the King's Chamber in the Egyptian Great Pyramid at Giza. Reid discovered that specific vowel sounds, when sung, create cymatic images that match Egyptian hieroglyphs.[3] That is amazing in itself, but more astounding is the knowledge that vowels sung by priests in the King's Chamber were thought to transport a soul into the netherworlds or alternative realms of reality.

The walls in the King's Chamber are composed of polished granite and when excited by sound, it is possible that the crystalline structure of the granite energetically released the encased geometry. Granite is composed mainly of quartz, mica, and feldspar. The building block of these materials is the silica tetrahedron, a geometric shape that will be very important as we continue to unfold the connection of geometry of sound throughout this book.

I believe that the sounds created within the chamber were used as a portal or bridge for living aspirants within the chamber to travel to other dimensions of consciousness.

Many experts believe that the King's Chamber was not a tomb but a religious ceremonial chamber, where sound was used to engender transcendental experiences and healing. My belief is that pure vowel sounds create coherent geometry and that this is one of the secrets that the Egyptian priests utilized in their healing rituals.

Ancient Greece

In ancient Greece, music was recognized for its healing qualities. Aristotle (323–373 B.C.E.), in his famous book *De Anima*, wrote that "flute music could arouse strong emotions and purify the soul."[4]

Greek asclepeions, healing temples sacred to the god Asclepius, offered people solace, healing, and hope, similar to modern health centers devoted to holistic medical practices. Essentially, these temples were the first hospitals. Among other treatments, the physicians that worked within them used music as a therapy for the healing of diseases both spiritual and physical. In preparation for the healing, the patients prepared and cleansed themselves by eating special diets or fasting, bathing, exercising, receiving massages, and attending musical events.

The instruments used by the Greek physicians were flutes, lyres, and zithers. Some of the great healing sound prescriptions they used were the musical modes. These are diatonic scales arranged with different half steps and whole steps per octave. It was believed that each of these modes carried specific vibrations and frequencies that had a profound effect on the patient and illness. And each mode was thought to have specific healing quality. For example, if a person was depressed, a physician might suggest that the patient listen to a lute playing in the Dorian mode, which is the scale from D to D containing a minor third and a major seventh.[5]

There are seven basic modes that can be played on the piano to be heard. For example, to hear an Aeolian mode, begin on the note A and play only white notes up to the higher note of A. You will have covered an octave. The modes are as follows.

- Aeolian is A–A
- Locrian is B–B
- Ionian is C–C
- Dorian is D–D
- Phrygian is E–E
- Lydian is F–F
- Mixolydian is G–G

Ionian philosopher Pythagoras (570–495 B.C.E.) felt that harmony in music was the immediate prerequisite for beauty. Sound and architecture were both recognized by Pythagoras as beautiful only when their parts were in harmonious balance. Pythagoras believed that "good and beauty" in pure form are musical. Beauty, he postulated, is harmony reflecting in the world of form.[6]

Of deep interest to me is the fact that Pythagoras spent twenty-three years in Egypt studying with the priesthood and was ultimately initiated into its deepest mysteries. He also spent time in India studying with Brahmin priests prior to opening his own mystery school in Greece. Perhaps he came to know the mystery of the Hindu *ragas* while in India. These are specific Indian scales used to induce various emotional states. It is well known that within the Pythagorean school, music was played for the students at the beginning of every day and also as a conclusion to the day's lessons, much like Indian musicians play ragas to greet the rising sun and the descent of night.

Ancient India

Ancient Indian ragas grew out of the principles of sacred sound. Ragas are still played today—a living artform. There are specific sound prescriptions for each time of day and for different emotions and spiritual states of being. Each prescription is based on specific scales and *talas* (rhythmic beat patterns). These were played on the veena (a stringed instrument), the sarangi venu (flute), and the mridanga or tabla (a pair of drums). Also, part of the musical tonal fabric was the well-known sitar, which was added as a stringed instrument during the sixteenth century.

The timeless principles of sacred sound are described in sacred Hindu scriptures, such as the Vedas and the Upanishads (1200–400 B.C.E.) Those sacred sources tell us that music, both vocal and instrumental, is divine in origin and closely linked with gods and goddesses. The goddess Saraswati, divine patron of music, is always shown with a veena in her hand. Brahma, creator of the universe, is always shown playing hand cymbals. Vishnu, the preserver, blows a conch shell; and his sacred descendant, Krishna, plays the flute. Shiva, the transformer or destroyer, in his depiction as Nataraja, plays the damaru drum to initiate the dance of creation. It seems that we have an entire orchestra represented by the gods and their beloved instruments. Maybe the emerging secret that is coming forward is that all divine energy is expressed in sound.

Each of these beloved instruments was thought of as a tool to evoke Nada-Brahman, the sacred, eternal sound represented by the syllable OM. *Nada* means "tone." *Brahman* is the unity that lies behind diversity. This sound was believed to bring the known universe into being—to bring matter into being from divine impulse.

Nada-Brahman, or OM, appears in musical writings as the foundation and wellspring of music. Yoga texts use the term OM to describe the musical and inner sounds heard in deep meditation. Nada refers to the cosmic sound, which can be unmanifested or manifested. Since Brahman, or God presence, pervades the entire universe, including the human soul, the concept of sacred sound as Nada-Brahman expresses the connection between the earthly realm and the divine realm.

The musical scales known as ragas are said to be just as timeless as the Brahman presence. Each raga expresses a specific *rasa* (mood or flavor) and can, when heard, generate those same feelings within both the listener and the performer.[7] When those feelings are directed toward the Divine, the result is a higher soul expression, as within Brahman, all is one. Musicians in India have a saying: "Through *svara* (musical notes), *Ishvara* (spiritual inspiration) is realized."[8]

Ancient Tibet

The Tibetan Buddhist rituals of sacred communion use sound more as an accompaniment to ceremony than as the focus of ceremony. Instruments used in ceremony include trumpets, gongs, cymbals, and bowls. The Dungchen, a long trumpet, is known for its incredibly resonant, deep sound, which is rich in overtones, not unlike those found in the sound of a gong, which is also used. Also present are bells and metal singing bowls, which are hammered from a combination of seven metals. When combined, these metals produce mystical sounds that are known to create trance-like states in listeners.

The metal singing bowls of Tibet are distinctly recognized as part of the landscape of meditative Tibetan music. They have a different sound than the quartz crystal singing bowls that seem to be more popular in the United States. As a sound therapist, I have found the metal bowls more difficult to play than the quartz singing bowls; however, many of my clients seem to prefer the sound and effect of the metal bowls.

Perhaps the most well-known musical instrument in the rituals of Tibetan Buddhism is the human voice—singing sacred chants. Most notable of performers are the throat singers of Tuva who train to sing two or three pitches at the same time. They do this by singing a fundamental pitch and then, through manipulation of resonant spaces in the mouth and throat, produce the overtones to the fundamental pitch. I have actually learned this technique and can outline the overtone series to a sung fundamental pitch.

Interestingly, my ancestral tree goes back to the Mongolian Yakut tribe who practice this type of singing. Perhaps this is why I found it so easy to learn the technique of overtone singing?

In any case, this type of singing produces powerful lower resonances layered with much higher overtones (or pitches) creating a melodic line. The droning sound effect is hypnotic. Its reported healing effects are attributed to the combination of paired pitches—the highest of which continue into the ultrasound range above human hearing.

We know that each organ within the human body has its own resonant frequency or pitch. In a healthy state, the frequency of the organ is coherent and not distorted. If the organ or body part is "out of tune" and operating at a less than optimal level, sickness may occur. The sounds of coherent frequencies with the overtones present in overtone singing can return the body to a state of health or return to harmony.

Ancient Aboriginal Australia

The indigenous people of Australia have a culture that extends back 40,000 years. Only recently have they had contact with the outside world. Their culture is spiritual and well ordered. Their rituals and life rhythms are unchanging in that their spiritual ancestors instructed them to follow a set pattern necessary to maintain the world. The many different types of instruments they use in ceremony are believed to continue the physical, worldly state of the *Dreaming,* their concept to describe the whole of Aboriginal life and culture and the landscape in which they live.

The didgeridoo, a wind instrument that originated in northern Australia, is now played in communities throughout the continent. Didgeridoo is perhaps the most well-known of the Aboriginal instruments. It has a resonant, deep pitch that can vary as the player alters his vocal tract space and lip pressure. Many times, a didgeridoo player will add his own vocal sound as part of the acoustics produced by the instrument. Its sound is not unlike the gong in that numerous frequencies and overtones accompany the fundamental pitch. This instrument has been popularized around the world by sound healers.

The percussion instruments of clap sticks and seed rattles are also popular, along with flat rocks and sticks of wood. In some areas, shells and leaves are tied together and laced around the ankles of ceremonial dancers to produce percussive sounds when dancing. Interestingly, we find this tradition in Africa as well. Less familiar an instrument is the ceremonial drum, used mainly by women.

Many of the sacred ceremonies are reserved for just the men and are closely guarded. No person, other than the elders of the community, is allowed to participate or observe.

Ancient Africa

Traditional African music used in sacred contexts is a combination of drumming and singing and chanting. Taking place in communal ceremonies, members of the community, overcome by forces brought forth by the rhythmic drumming and chanting, are excited to the point of going into meditative trance.

One such religious ceremony, from Cameroon, is the Okuyi, which is practiced by several Bantu ethnic groups. Its purpose is to call forth the spirit of sacred deities or respected ancestors. The rhythms and instruments the musicians play depend upon the region. Members of the community can embody and channel the energy of a deity or respected ancestor. They use ritual movements to deepen their altered state of consciousness. Once in a trance, they can be connected to the advice and counsel from the discarnate deity or ancestor and pass this information along to the rest of the community.

It has been known that drumming can induce altered states of consciousness, but the science of why this creates these altered states has only recently been discovered and little is yet understood. I believe the altered state is induced through two means: forced brainwave states and sensory dampening of the part of the brain that is responsible for physical awareness.

Let us first discuss *forced brainwave states*. In part, the African shaman's technique relies on influencing the fundamental, natural behavior of the brain.

Brain activity and brainwave states are measured as electrical impulses (frequencies). The speed of these impulses determines the individual's state of consciousness. The four basic levels of brainwaves and states of consciousness are delta, theta, alpha, and beta. Our brainwave state can be influenced by external sound or light stimulus. If the stimuli are approximately four beats per second, this will drive the brain into a theta state of consciousness.

The slowest brainwave state is delta, whose signature is sound frequencies up to 4 Hz. A hertz is one cycle per second. This first state is associated with unconsciousness and the deepest level of sleep.

The second level of consciousness, theta, occurs when the speed of brainwaves is between 4 and 8 Hz. This state is where hallucinations and imagery take place and is the state we enter when we meditate, have trancelike experiences, or go on shamanic journeys rich in mental imagery.

The third state of consciousness is alpha, encompassing brainwave activity in the range between 8 and 13 Hz. Alpha is a relaxed, daydreamy state where we are aware of the external world and feel relaxed.

The fourth level of consciousness is beta. Beta occurs when the speed of brainwaves is between 13 and 30 Hz. This is our normal, wakeful state of being. High beta exists above 30 Hz and is associated with manic states and feelings of euphoria.[9]

Research on gamma waves, which lie above 40 Hz, is only just coming forward, as the ability to measure this wave state can only be measured with digital electroencephalogram (EEG) machines. It is thought that the gamma state signals whole brain evolvement, enhanced learning, and perceptions of unity.

Research that supports how drumming (external sound) can alter consciousness in the form of auditory driving is fairly recent. I have experienced this altered state many times within the contexts of shamanic journeys. To journey, a person lies down and closes his eyes—typically while listening to steady drumming. It usually takes about five minutes to enter into the altered states of low alpha and theta, wherein the colors and images become vivid and distinct. There is also a contextual meaning to the images that does not seem to be available in the higher brainwave states of the high alpha and beta states.

The science is now showing that sensory stimulus travels to the base of the brain called the reticular activating system (RAS). This part of the brain controls brainwave activity and governs which state is needed to meet the consciousness demands of the moment. For example, if a high beta state is needed to escape danger, the RAS would initiate that state; and conversely, if a low alpha, relaxed state is needed to return to homeostasis, the RAS could return the body to that state with appropriate and effective direction.

The second way the altered state is achieved through drumming is to create a disturbed self-processing phenomenon. This is called *sonic forcing*. In continuous and strong drumming there is a breakdown of sensory integration in the temporal parietal junction within the brain. When the brain gets stimulated repeatedly by sound, it eventually habituates, shuts down, and no longer responds to sensory and physical signals within the body. The result of this is that the subject has the sensation of traveling to different environments in another body. The real physical body no longer responds to the surrounding physical and sensory environment. Out-of-body experiences such as these are common in the presence of massive drumming stimulation. For indigenous peoples, this method of slipping into trance is valued as a mystical state wherein an individual may commune with spirits and journey into the altered realms of reality.

Medieval Europe

Gregorian chanting is an unaccompanied monophonic (one vocal line) form of sacred Roman Catholic music that emerged in western and central Europe during the ninth and tenth centuries. It is often said that Pope Saint Gregory I invented Gregorian chant. It is more likely, however, that he simply collected chants by various composers within the Church and collated them. The vocal form is unlike any music in Europe prior to the ninth century in that the melodic lines soar and sweep, with extended vowel sounds, creating an auric impression of spin.

The genesis of plainchant in the West probably came from early Jewish chants used in religious services. Having sung both cantorial chant for Jewish High Holiday services and also Roman Catholic chants within masses, I can say that the similarities are evident to me. But Roman Catholic chanting is much more melismatic—meaning, a single syllable of text is sung while vocal movement covers several notes. Roman Catholic chanting also covers a greater range of notes than Jewish chanting does.

One of the most notable composers of Gregorian chant was Hildegard von Bingen, an extraordinary woman who became the abbess of a German Benedictine monastery. She entered the monastery at the age of fourteen and was experiencing visions at that early age. She kept these hidden from the Church's knowledge until her early forties. Urged by the light within her visions, she was commanded to write down what she heard and saw during these experiences. Her luminous chants came after this directive from her divine source. Her "compositions" are unique and breathtakingly beautiful in that they are improvisatory in feeling and scope. For me, the effect of hearing and singing these chants is transformative. One can easily lose track of time and space as the notes wrap sonic light around the listener and singer.

As was customary for music composed during this period, there are no tempo markings and no rhythmic notations in the compositions of Hildegard von Bingen. Hence, the vocal lines seem to cross into a "no time" space and the listener can easily move into a trance state. I can only imagine the benefit of hearing these chants throughout the day as was customary for the nuns within the monastery where they originated.

Ancient North America

Native North Americans used techniques of drumming in much the same way that African shamans used them: to commune with ancestors and receive messages from spirits. Also, to prepare for the hunt or a battle.

It is known that drumming has the ability to shut down left-brain activity. The left-brain is the part of the brain responsible for logical, linear, and analytical thinking. When its activity quiets, the right-brain can become fully active and engaged. The right-brain is the part of the brain that is thought to be responsible for visual creativity and gestalt awareness.

Drums have been used worldwide for millennia to ready warriors to go into battle. Who can forget the scene in the movie *Braveheart*, depicting the rebellion of the Scots against the rule of England in the thirteenth-century, in which the Scots, against massive odds, were preparing to rush into battle with the English troops? The drums in that movie scene were deafening in hopes that the infantry would not think or analyze, and perhaps think twice about the slaughter that was about to occur.

Another technique that has been used to put warriors into altered states before a battle is *photon forcing*. This is the technique of using flickering lights to alter brainwaves and usher in theta consciousness. Dancing around a flickering fire is a perfect example of that kind of photon forcing. The brain, through photon entrainment, moves into altered states. After participating in nighttime ceremonies, a battle facing a Native warrior would have taken on a mythic quality.

Ancient Central and South America

The indigenous peoples of Central and South America have used sound, song, and rhythm as a bridge into the altered realms of consciousness for millennia. Typically, the medicinal plants of the region are used as part of the ceremonies to create this bridge with the additional stimulating qualities of sound. I have experienced ceremonies where a drink prepared from the plant ayahuasca (sometimes called the vine of the soul) is drunk. I have direct knowledge of the *icaros,* magical songs sung during the ceremony by native Shipibo shamans. The intention for these sacred ceremonies is to gain understanding of life issues, disease, relationships, and life purpose. They have been used for thousands and thousands of years as a central part of their indigenous spiritual practice.

The following is an account from my time in Peru spent at a sanctuary deep in the Amazon jungle. This account of the sacred ceremonies and the influence of sound and song comes from my direct experience.

Ceremonies in the Amazon Jungle

To prepare to participate in the sacred medicine ceremony, it is necessary to have clarity of purpose. The ceremonies are offered as opportunities for deep soul work and subconscious exploration. Many people come to the Amazon to heal either physical conditions or mental trauma. I felt called by the deep longing to know and experience my divine self. The preparation for this type of journey takes at least two weeks of adhering to a strict diet of just vegetables, eggs, rice, and fruit. This clears the body of waste and chemical toxins. It was made clear to me that the only medication I could ingest during the month prior to the ceremony was aspirin. It would prove a challenge for me, as I experience frequent migraines, but my will was fierce. I resolved to "do what it takes."

I arrived at the sanctuary five pounds lighter than when I began the cleansing diet, full of anticipation and hope. My intention for this first ceremony was to understand the icaros that would be sung by the shaman watching over our group. I wanted to learn the genesis of these songs and what musical form, scales, and keys were customarily used. I was pleased to receive much information along those lines.

Although it may seem like a bizarre claim, a distinct voice is heard within the ceremony, which has been identified as the feminine energy of the plant. Thus, many refer to the plant medicine as Mother Ayahuasca. I heard her voice speaking to me in my mind and it was not my own voice.

To set the stage, the sanctuary in which the ceremonies are held is a *maloca,* a round, ancestral building with a very high thatched roof. All the participants come into the maloca to sit on a specifically chosen mat that will be their "home" for the ceremonies planned for the week. In totality, I participated in four. These mats circle the perimeter of the maloca wall like flower petals.

To begin the ceremony, an hour of meditation proceeds for centering and clarifying the intentions that are to be stated to Mother Ayahuasca before the drinking of the brew. The vine is found deep in the jungle and the energy of its brew guides supplicants into many memories and profound awareness, which ultimately heal and enlighten them.

Sometimes Mother Ayahuasca throws a tough love approach at the pilgrims. I understood I might be confronted and was ready for whatever she gave me. I knew that in my current lifetime, my soul has chosen to integrate many aspects of my life with my past lives as well. It has been my soul's choice. However, I was not fully prepared to experience as many past lives of trauma and fear as I did. How could I have known?

Mother Aya let me experience previous incarnations and, with great love, showed me lessons my soul had learned from those lives. I must say that many were traumatic with painful deaths that were not uncommon in our history as a species. But I did not run away from the lessons shown to me and finally came to the profound understanding and gratitude for the past life and even the excruciating death. There was meaning in it all.

After an hour of meditation, the shaman entered the maloca and the ceremony began with each of us (there were eighteen in total) drinking the medicine from a small cup. It tasted nasty, but I hoped the benefit would far outweigh a momentary "ugh." I drank and returned to my mat to await the first reaction, which for me was intense colors and patterns moving before my eyes.

Entering a stage of visions and colors, I saw a brilliant mandala appear before me. It was orange and yellow, with colors that moved and circulated. The mandala, as I later learned, was the pattern known as the *flower of life*, which is composed of seven circles overlapping within a larger circle. This pattern has appeared in spiritual art all over the world for thousands of years. It has been embroidered in the shamanic art of the Amazon as well. Having subsequently studied it, I feel that it represents patterns of nature that are webbed into the space-time fabric of the quantum field. It is an emblem of sacred geometry.

Because my intention for the first ceremony was to understand the power of the icaros, I listened to the singing with musician's ears and quickly realized that they are built on a pentatonic scale, which is composed of five notes: E, F-sharp, A, B, and C-sharp. The intervals of this scale are the same as those between the black notes on the piano. All the notes can sound together, and nothing sounds dissonant to the ear.

The fact that the pentatonic scale was used, and all the notes could be sung together without dissonance, became very clear to me when five shaman sometimes would be singing their own individual icaros simultaneously, while the tonal fabric remained harmonious. The sound was stunning in beauty. Occasionally, the melodies of various singers would touch on other notes, but the main structure was built around the pentatonic scale.

I began to see different patterns emerge with each icaros as colors and geometric patterns wafted in the air before me.

I saw the music with my eyes open. I also realized that the structure of the space-time fabric is revealed in shapes and pattern. The icaros were manipulating that fabric and hence the energy I felt in the maloca. Amazing.

In my mind, I questioned where the pentatonic scale came from and Mother Aya said that it is built into the human voice as the overtone series. It is integral to us. We are all carriers of this pattern. Whenever we speak or sing, we are creating this pattern in the air.

The overtone series follows a very set pattern that always begins with a fundamental pitch. If our fundamental pitch is C, the overtones (webbed frequencies within the fundamental pitch) are C, an octave; G, a fifth; C, a perfect fourth; E, a major third; G, a minor third; B-flat, another minor third; and C, a major second.

The overtone series will be discussed in depth in Chapter 4.

Pentatonic scales are present in all the music of the ancient cultures and grew naturally out of the human singing and sounding voice. It is quite easy to sound the overtone series with your own voice by manipulating the resonating chambers within your mouth. The overtone series clearly emerges. This scale has been part of us from the beginning due to the structure of our physiology.

As the hours in the ceremony continued to pass, my chin began quivering and I felt that I needed to open my mouth. Mother Ayahuasca entered my throat, opened it, and deepened my breath. Very often, her energy can take the shape of a snake or jaguar. In this case, she was a snake and I could feel her energy descending into my body. I was not afraid, as I trusted her. She went to my feet and began to shake me like a snake and used my hands and arms to point at vines wafting in the air above me as she gave me her instruction.

She said, "Your hands are my hands. Use them to heal. To call on me, just sing my tone." That tone was an E, which all the shamans I heard sing used as their vocal home base. It is also the pitch of the chakra in the solar plexus. The color resonant with this is a saffron orange-yellow, like the color of the robes worn by Tibetan monks.

Continuing, she said, "I live in you now. I wrote the songs you composed. Take this knowledge into your world and use it to bring the ones who can hear to knowledge and awareness. My songs are bridges to the soul. I am compassion. I am the feminine energy coming into the world. I have had many faces from many cultures and times throughout history. This is only one such time. You have carried my energy and been killed for it, but it is all part of the evolution of your species."

"You carry me now. When you sound or sing, you are the voice of the divine feminine. Your music is my music. Take my voice into music for your world as my voice is compassion, caring, and nurturing. You are daughter to the Mother. I shake you to fully integrate this sound energy into each cell of your body."

While under the influence of Ayahuasca, none of this information seemed alarming or strange. It made perfect sense. I knew that I was not special in the sense that only I was given this knowledge. This knowledge is available and can be used by all who recognize that the energy of love heals. After the ceremony was over and the effects of the brew began to dissipate, my recall of the information was crystal clear. Everything said to me was remembered in detail.

I ultimately went back to my hut to sleep. During the early morning hours, I woke up shaking and breathing fast and shallow like I do in ceremony. I woke up to *know* that F-sharp is the portal to the folded reality that contains the intertwined geometry of all two-dimensional and three-dimensional shapes—the Platonic solids. Quantum physics suggests that there are many realms of folded or hidden reality, which lie in potential within the energetic field of possibilities.

From previous research, I understood that within the F-sharp (F#) pitch resides the geometry of the tetrahedron, which has folded within it all geometric patterns. I had been told that with the repeating toning of F# and the playing of pitches, F#, A-sharp (A#), and C-sharp (C#) with quartz crystal singing bowls, the crown chakra will open energetically. It responds to the constant activation of the F# frequency. The process, I was told, is to tone the pitch F# while listening to the crystal singing bowls play F#, A#, C#, and then experience the silence following the tones to integrate the energy.

That morning in Peru, while still in my mosquito-netted bed, I listened to the bird calls in the jungle and realized that they ALL center around F or F#. One bird sang his song maybe fifty times outside my window. His sweet song was the melody of E, F#, F#, C#, F#. Occasionally he would throw in F#, G#, G#, C#, F#.

Another bird would repeat F# over and over.

My thoughts were that they birds were just giving voice to the frequencies in the unified or quantum field of energetic possibilities, the sound was the energetic field made audible. They were singing the unity of all. It was magnificent.

Ancient Roots of Afro-American Gospel Music

In reflection on traditional African music, it should be noted that the music of tribal peoples was used in ceremony and filled with specific purposes that addressed the flow of their community activities and daily lives. They performed songs and dances that appealed to the gods for rain, for agricultural and personal fertility, and for successful warfare. This African approach to music was closely aligned with the approach of the Native North Americans who used music in much the same way. Both ancient cultures used drumming, rhythmic dancing, and singing as a way to celebrate the passing of seasons, honor deities, and enter altered states of consciousness.

Music that referred to and celebrated secular life was not existent in Africa. As the transatlantic Portuguese slave trade flourished from the sixteenth through the nineteenth centuries, the suffering of the people captured and sold into slavery from Western and Central Africa was profound. It is estimated that 10–12 million Africans were brought to the Americas by traders. It is still difficult for me to accept that the human species is capable of such brutality and degradation as was present in the slave trade. However, it happened, and the Africans subjugated to such suffering had little to comfort themselves save their music.

As an aside, in tracing my genetic lineage, I have found that I have ancestral DNA from West Africa that goes only five generations back. To imagine any of us as separate from one another is an illusion both in terms of our subtle energy and in our ancestral history. We are one. I can clearly imagine the suffering of my human family.

During this period of fear, confusion, and trauma, the enslaved Africans and their descendants sang the songs of their musical ancestry to connect them to the remaining shreds of their tribal and community life. It is from these roots that modern-day gospel music was born. This totally new style of music was created by mixing the African traditions of harmony and call and response with a strong, rhythmic pulse.

In later years, the European traditions of harmony and European musical instruments, namely the piano, were incorporated into the rich heritage of gospel music.

I have been fascinated and drawn to the call and response form of the African traditions. Typically, one voice sings a very short musical phrase and then the group echoes the same phrase. Sometimes, the leader varies the call, but the response is always the same melody and words. As a response to the strong rhythmic component, the group and leader may fall into a simple dance, which connects the participants in both melody and rhythm and movement. In this way, a mental and spiritual connection is created that allows the group to enjoy and establish deep connection.

Thus, the "strength in numbers" phenomenon was established that continues today in gospel music. During gospel singing, there is a cessation of analytical thinking and the participants flow into a state of just being and experiencing joy in the moment. It is a form of ecstatic flow, which I have experienced personally at the Agape International Spiritual Center, a new thought church located in Culver City, California. Members of the church come from all walks of life and the feeling within the church is of unconditional love and compassion for all. Michael Bernard Beckwith is the visionary minister who created and formed this gathering of beautiful people. I was moved to tears as I felt wrapped in loving sound during the call and response singing. It is a very powerful and joyful form of music.

....

TWO

COMMON ELEMENTS IN SACRED HEALING MUSIC

To explore the realm of sacred music, we must first define it. From its name, we can surmise that this style of music reflects the ideas and values of the religious institutions in Europe. Partly, this is true. But to only limit our thinking to the European model of sacred music constricts our view. Even so, let us initially investigate this narrow view.

The first music to be recognized within the Roman Catholic Church was monophonic chant. The Church supported and accepted this kind of chanting within the mass prior to the fourteenth century, or the inception of the Renaissance. The name *Gregorian chant* comes from the fact that Pope Gregory I found this type of monophonic singing so supportive to the mass that he collected and cataloged the liturgical chants still used today.

The next huge revolution within sacred European music came at the dawn of the Renaissance (circa 1400), when two-part harmony, then three-part harmony and even more complex harmonies emerged within the musical landscape of sacred music. The glorious period of Baroque music, which includes the music of close contemporaries Johann Sebastian Bach (1685–1750) and George Frideric Handel (1685–1759), was about to offer humanity aural landscapes of breathtaking beauty.

I adhere to the belief that music reflects the collective consciousness of a culture, so to understand a culture the first place to go is to its music. From a historical point of view, we can discern that Europeans were emerging into a more evolved expression of thought and consciousness, as the music that infused their culture reflected this expansion. No longer were human ears capable of only absorbing one vocal line. We were being bathed in glorious harmony from many voices and instruments and varying rhythmic patterns. It was a banquet of many delights.

To enlarge our view now to encompass the global community, music has been used in ceremony from the beginning of our history as we lived and flourished in human community. To reserve the term *sacred* to European music exclusively would be a grave mistake. Sacred music is any that allows the spirit to express love and unity.

To be clear, all music does not lift the spirit to the same heights of love. Even so, I would not classify any music as *secular* or *profane*, just as I would not presume to classify any human with those labels. Those types of judgments catapult us into duality—a state of separation from one another. I believe music can help us develop greater understanding of one another and teach us compassion and empathy, so that we can bring those virtues into our daily lives and relationships.

How does music facilitate healing? There are many ways that it affects the mind, body, and soul. Some ways directly influence the physical body. Some ways, the bioenergetic body. And some, the subtler etheric body.

Let us take a more in-depth look at the entrainment of brainwaves and brainwave states. *Entrainment* is a phenomenon in which music affects us on a primal, unconscious level. Our bodies intuitively adjust to the rhythms of music in a phenomenon known as *brainwave entrainment.* Allow me to explain this from the perspective of the different brainwave states that dictate our subjective reality.

Let us revisit the five different brainwave states that are central to healing.

Lying above 40 Hz (or cycles per second), gamma brainwaves are the highest frequency possible for the human brain. The state of consciousness associated with gamma waves is peak concentration. They represent the brain's optimal functioning for cognitive activity. Many studies have been done to measure the brainwave of Tibetan monks deep in meditation and gamma waves were always present. The gamma state is characterized by unity consciousness or the perception of energetic reality. This frequency is an ultrasonic tone we cannot hear.

The frequency of beta brainwaves lies between 13–40 Hz. Interestingly, the pitch of 40 Hz is about an E. The beta state is characterized by a high level of alertness. The mind is sharp, focused, and makes connections quickly and easily. The neurons react quickly and efficiently, helping to achieve excellent mental performance.

The alpha state is a delightful and relaxed state of consciousness. It is induced when the frequency of the brainwaves is 8–12 Hz. All stress-reduction tools aim to put us in this brainwave state as it is essential to achieving relaxation and has positive physical benefits. Highly creative people, such as painters, musicians, and writers, are adept alpha wave producers. I find myself slipping into this state when I sing or compose. Light meditation or daydreaming signals the presence of the alpha state.

Alpha researcher, Joe Kamiya, Ph.D., at the University of Chicago, in his book *Biofeedback and Self-Control,* says, "Its pleasure may come from the fact that alpha represents something like letting go of anxieties."[1] This is a key definition, as anxiety produces the chemical cascade of cortisol and adrenaline that is detrimental to health if it is a chronic state.

Theta brainwave state, between 4 and 8 Hz, is the twilight state that is normally only experienced upon waking or drifting off to sleep. Mystical information is often received when we're in theta, which is the bridge between our subconscious and conscious minds. I experience this state in my meditation practice when I "return" to alpha state and wonder where I have been.

The delta state is the state of deep sleep. Delta waves are the slowest of all five brainwave frequencies and range from 0–4 Hz. Physical healing is facilitated in this state. It should be noted that if someone suffers from sleep deprivation, the physical healing process is severely compromised.

In recognizing how we can enter these various brainwave states, we can consider both rhythmic and light entrainment. I have tried specialized eyeglasses that pulse at a targeted rate to entrain my brain to enter a theta state. The glasses were effective, but my preference is binaural sound and rhythmic entrainment. Music with a strong beat stimulates brainwaves to synchronize with the beat. Faster rhythms increase alertness and focus, while slower beats encourage a relaxed, meditative state. These alterations in brainwaves influence the body via the autonomic nervous system, which governs involuntary functions like heart rate, blood pressure, breathing, and cortisol levels.

The sympathetic branch of the autonomic nervous system is designed to defend the body against danger and elicits the infamous fight-or-flight response. When the crisis has passed, the parasympathetic branch takes over again, and the body returns to healing. Music with slower rhythms has a profound effect on the nervous system and assists in keeping us in a healing mode instead of a defensive mode.

The parasympathetic nervous system, the vagus nerve response, and the attendant flow of neurochemicals helps us make the return to a healing state. We shall take an in-depth look at this restorative process in Chapter 7.

Because of the challenges inherent to modern life, many of us live in a state of continual sympathetic arousal. If you stay in a crisis-reaction mode, it means that stress hormones are wearing down your body. All your energy is going toward defense, and there's no opportunity for your body to rebuild, heal, and regenerate.

Music is one of the easiest, most immediate ways to produce the parasympathetic state of healing. We know that music with a slow tempo will calm the nervous system and encourage parasympathetic activity, as heart rate and breathing tend to synchronize to the beat of the music spontaneously. Studies have shown that a musical tempo of about seventy beats per minute is perfect because it mimics the average healthy heart.

There is another possibility we must consider as we review the healing effects of sound. Studying the phenomenon of sound made visible, research has revealed another astounding effect of sound frequencies: the creation of images in matter. We shall review the field of *cymatics* in depth later on in this book. Here I just want to say that it has been revealed how each pitch or frequency is encoded with a specific geometric pattern. This emerges when a specific sound frequency is applied to material such as sand on a brass plate or particulates in fluid.

Knowing that the physical body is 80 percent fluid, we can draw the conclusion that sound can produce either geometric coherence or geometric distortion in the physical body (and also the energetic biofield). Illness or disease is a distortion of that inherent, ordered geometry of frequency.

The eastern view is that life energy (*prana* or *chi*) flows within meridian patterns in the human body. Could it be that sound can stimulate the flow to reflect optimal health and through forced resonance restore the balanced order? In other words, by subjecting the physical, etheric, and subtle body energy to cohesive sound, could we not assist and facilitate a healthy flow of energy within the body? My belief is that this is how healing can occur. Where there is dense or "stuck" energy, a healing frequency can serve as an aid to health and energetic flow.

THREE

MUSICAL ELEMENTS OF HEALING SOUND

A s my research deepened, I recognized that common elements were emerging within the sacred music traditions. Certainly, the specific cultures would have different signatures, but numerous similarities started to come into focus. Let us explore those similarities.

Drone

Drones are sustained or continuous tones within a musical composition that establish a tonal center or carpet to accompany instruments or voices. A drone is the root note of a particular key. For example, in the key of C, the root pitch is C. As a drone is played or sounded vocally, the fifth note in the key (in this case, G) is often added to establish more harmonic context.

By consciously avoiding the major or minor third of the chord in the instrumental harmony, a musician or singer is free to explore both major and minor chords in their improvised melodic exploration above the drone to create aural interest. The effect of a drone is one of relaxation and a cessation of time, as time is created by distinct rhythm within the musical texture. Harmonies and vocal lines moving slowly above the drone further enhance the effect of relaxation and peace. Drones give the listener a feeling of stability and safety.

Classical East Indian music utilizes this technique, as does Irish bagpipe music.

Melodic and Harmonic Repetition

Examples of melodic and harmonic repetition are very clearly heard in the call and response form of singing first evident in African sacred music, where a leader sings a phrase that is then repeated back to them by the community. This form of music unites participants in common tones, common breath, and common movement, fostering connection and a sense of belonging. Unity is achieved through sound and movement. The result of this unity is health in mind and body, as we are a tribal species and flourish and prosper within any structure that bonds us. Singing of folk songs around a campfire was a common occurrence in my childhood both in our family backyard and at Girl Scout Camp. Although the call and response technique is not common in folk music, the same result of unity is achieved by the lusty group singing of the chorus of a song like "Home on the Range."

The present state of humanity is in jeopardy now as we are losing our ability to connect by sight, heart, and touch. We have been cast into an unknown land of disconnection and alienation. We yearn for the feeling of coming home, which, at a base level, I believe has to do with the human need for connection, one to another. What better way to feel this place of home than to sing and move together?

Repetition in melody and harmony gives the brain security because it eliminates the need for constantly scanning for the proverbial lion in the grasses. The brain can relax in its knowing that there is a predictable pattern it can recognize in the tonal landscape.

Rhythm

Rhythm is the master facilitator for brainwave entrainment and distinct brainwave states. To enter the desired state is as easy as listening to a drum beating out the signature beats per minute of the targeted brainwave. Drumming circles are magical places to experience this phenomenon. Typically, participants bring their own drums and a facilitator can create any number of ways to proceed with the circle. Many times, there is a designated solid beat drummer who establishes a rhythm. Other drummers create patterns that revolve around that specific beat. Other times, there is no specific direction given to the drummers, but eventually a group pattern emerges, which is magic in itself. Out of chaos comes pattern.

I have experienced drumming in shamanic journey circles with the shaman both drumming and leading the group through a journey of visions described by mental pictures. On these occasions, I slipped into a deep alpha state where in my mind's eye I "saw" many magical things, visions that imparted information full of deep knowing.

Rhythm has been used by our culture to create varying states, as among them military cohesiveness. I am reminded of pictures of thousands of soldiers marching to drums, totally united in mind, body, and soul. This unity was created by rhythm. Rhythm can shut down the analytical side of the brain and send people into a land of "no thought" as evidenced by the incessant rhythm used in dance clubs filled with dancers blissed into a state of nothingness and movement. I experienced this in a workshop with Gabrielle Roth, founder of 5Rhythms, a dancer who introduced therapeutic movement and dance to nondancers like myself. During the dance I attended, hundreds of people in a hotel ballroom were moving dynamically to very strong rhythmic pulses. I reached a state wherein my body took over and my mind just enjoyed observing the dance. I was not aware at all of thought or self-consciousness. I simply was along for the magnificent ride of movement for movement's sake. It was fabulous.

Rhythm in different meters, such as 3/4 time, 4/4 time, 6/8 time, or any number of other rhythmic possibilities, has different effects on the listener or the music makers. The meter is determined by the number of notes played or sung per measure of music. These patterns are easily recognizable, even to the non-musician. We all know the comfort of a lullaby, for instance, which is always in 3/4 time, is the meter of a waltz. The 1-2-3 . . . 1-2-3 . . . 1-2-3 repetition is hypnotic and encourages a swaying motion.

Three-quarter-time is more static and flowing in nature than 4/4 time, which is 1-2-3-4. . . 1-2-3-4 . . . 1-2-3-4, a meter that suggests a steady walking or running forward movement.

When music has no perceptible rhythm, the result is deep relaxation because the brain cannot anticipate the pattern and therefore releases any rhythmic expectation.

Melodic Intervals

To move further into our study of musical healing, let us explore the world of musical *intervals,* a concept that describes the harmonic relationship between two notes. Musical intervals can play a profound role in our healing as the intervals encourage energetic movement in our consciousness. Numerous studies have shown that each musical interval, such as a third or a fifth chord, invokes a specific emotional reaction in the listener. The most important intervals for healing purposes are listed below.

For the sake of comprehension, I am providing examples using the scale Do-Re-Mi-Fa-Sol-La-Ti-Do, just like in the song "Doe, a Deer" from *The Sound of Music.* I will also give you musical examples from familiar songs to help you discern the intervals. When there are mentions of an overtone series, I am referring to natural harmonics or pitches that are part of any sound which color the tone to give it its unique timbre. The fundamental pitch (the one clearly heard) is just the first note in the series. There are many more that lie above that fundamental, some being stronger, and some weaker.

Octave (for example, Do–Do). When two pitches are sounded together an octave apart, the higher pitch is twice the frequency of the lower pitch. They are the same note, eight notes apart. This interval suggests rest, stability, home, and grounding. An octave is the first overtone in the overtone series and thus is very familiar to the ear.

A musical example is the interval between the first two notes of "Somewhere Over the Rainbow" from *The Wizard of Oz.*

Perfect Fifth (Do–Sol). This interval is five notes apart. The second (higher) pitch is the second harmonic in the overtone series. This interval suggests stability, balance, completeness, and joy. The fifth is present in many folk songs because of its familiarity and placement in the series; it is the second overtone.

A musical example is the interval between the second and third notes in the children's tune "Twinkle, Twinkle Little Star."

Perfect Fourth (Do–Fa). This interval is four notes apart and suggests serenity and openness. Very often, this interval is used in trumpet calls and horn calls. The interval does have a harmonic tension. The mind wants it to resolve the tension within the interval by moving one note down to the third for resolution or move up one note to the fifth for stability.

Musical examples are the first notes of "Here Comes the Bride" (melody from Richard Wagner's *Lohengrin*) or the late eighteenth-century hymn "Amazing Grace."

Major Third (Do–Mi). This interval is sonic stability itself. When we hear this interval, it suggests joy, happiness, resolution, and peace. The number three has been reflected in many aspects of divinity and creation. Thirds are used liberally in Mexican folk music such as is performed by mariachi bands. The ability to vocally harmonize with thirds is also a popular musical technique in barbershop quartets.

Musical examples are "Kumbaya" and "From the Halls of Montezuma."

Major Second (Do–Re). This interval of two neighboring notes played simultaneously or in succession can be dissonant. It contains within its harmonic sound the need to resolve to either a unison (same sound) which is the neighboring lower note or up a note to create a third which would be the neighboring higher note.

Musical examples are the first two notes of "Doe, a Deer" and "Frère Jacques."

Major Sixth (Do–La). This interval is perhaps the most etheric of all the intervals. There is no tension within the interval to move or resolve to a lower or higher note. There is no emotional heaviness or bitterness to the interval, although it can express sweet sadness.

A musical example is the first two notes of "My Bonnie Lies over the Ocean."

Major Seventh (Do–Ti). This interval is a fascinating aural example of sweet resolution. It is called the *leading tone interval* because it holds great energy in its need to resolve to the root tone. It desires a movement to wholeness/oneness and therefore is used often in new age healing music. To hold the major seventh in a melodic line before resolving to the root pitch causes tension in the mind of the listener. I have used this interval abundantly in my compositions as a way to hold the ear in expectation, without a rhythmic form. Holding the seventh pitch within a melodic line creates a floating feeling. Some composers have labeled this interval the *healing interval* and I concur.

A musical example is the tune from *South Pacific* "Bali Hai."

Diminished Fifth, or "Tritone" (Do–flatted Sol). This is an interval of great dissonance, which does not rest in the ear until its resolution to the major fifth (the upper neighboring note.) In the Medieval period in Europe, it was called the *devil's interval* because it was thought to be able to summon demons by opening a sonic portal. I love this interval because it evokes a suspended feeling in a melodic line in much the same way that the major seventh interval does. It carries a sweet longing in its energy.

Musical examples are "Maria" from *West Side Story* or the theme song from *The Simpsons.*

After pondering and experiencing these intervals both as a composer and as a performer, one simple question arose in my mind: *Why do these intervals affect us so profoundly?* It then occurred to me that the musical overtone series follows a set pattern. The overtone series are the unheard harmonics or pitches present in every sound. Some of the harmonics are weaker and some stronger. A person's voice has a unique quality because of the overtone array present in an individual's sound. We can easily identify a person on the phone by the sound of his or her voice. Each voice is unique because of the overtone or harmonic signature.

The first five tones in the series always outline an octave, a perfect fifth, and a major third. Those three notes sounded together are known as a major triad. Sing the first three notes of "Kumbaya," and you are hearing these three pitches in succession which outline the major third triad.

We associate the major triad sound with a choir of angels singing, trumpets announcing the arrival of royalty, and the ultimate chord of consonance and stability. It is very much beloved for its harmonic properties by listeners.

In my compositions I have used major triads and intentional repetitions of major seventh intervals in both the chordal structure and the melodic line. The suspended energy created by the major seventh yearns for resolution into the octave. Many compositions have been written of late that use this interval, as it energetically calls the ear and the body into *consonance,* which is the state of health, and musically, of resolution.

Musical Keys

Another aspect of music is the key in which a piece of music or a song is written, which goes hand in hand with the emotional response to that key. For example, music written in the key of C is said to reflect feelings of purity and innocence, while music written in the key of F minor suggests feelings of despair and sadness.

I am a pianist and I know that playing a song in the key of C major is much different than playing the same piece in the key of D major. The additional sharps needed to perform the key of D seem to brighten the sound. Keys with flats in the key signature tend to soften the sound and make it richer and warmer. For this very reason, gospel music and rhythm and blues music are typically written in keys with flats.

For our purposes, below I will list the keys and associated emotional signatures that are fairly common in vocal and piano literature.

- C major (no flats or sharps), completely pure key, sounds of innocence, simplicity

- G major (one sharp in this key), key of triumph over difficulty
- D major (two sharps), key of triumph, hallelujah, victory rejoicing ("Hallelujah Chorus," anyone?)
- F major (one flat), plaintive
- B flat major (two flats), magnificent and joyful
- E flat major (three flats), strong devotion
- D minor (one flat), melancholy, gentleness
- A minor (no sharps or flats), tenderness of character
- E minor (one sharp), declaration of love, a few tears, resolution
- B minor (two sharps), patience, bending to divine will

I concur that this interpretation is partly subjective; however, there may be some universal truth to the description of these emotional responses that cannot be measured or accurately described, which lies below conscious awareness.

Melodies

Musical melodies are treasures troves if we scratch away at the surface of what makes a melody pleasing, healing, irritating, or any of the myriad emotional responses we have to melody. It is my belief that melodies which express joy are the most healing. Why do we like some melodies and some we do not? Partly for personal reasons. But let's see if we can also draw some universal truths.

Melodies that use a limited range of notes are more peaceful and calming as they do not challenge either voice or ear.

I am also reminded of the melodies of the Gregorian chants with their slow progression of notes. Melodies that have long melodic phrases tend to slow the heartbeat as the heart entrains to the longer phrases. Long phrases relax us.

Conversely, shorter phrases enliven the heart.

We tend to enjoy melodies where the notes are reasonably close together with a variety of lovely, harmonious intervals between the notes. If the rhythm mirrors the tempo of speech, all the better. It seems that if melodies are similar to sentences our brains are designed to listen to, we feel comfortable with the melody.

Melodies can express different emotions. For example, melodies in minor keys seem to carry darker, sadder emotion and melodies in major keys are brighter.

Interestingly, if a melody covers just a few notes, it is recognized as sad—like the monotone voice with which a depressed person would speak. In contrast, a happy person uses a larger range in their speaking voice and pattern. Happy music and melodies reflect this same pattern . . . their melodies use larger intervals over a wider range.

Harmony

Harmony is formed with two or more pitches are sounded at the same time to form chords. The word *harmony* has also been used to describe people or nations in a state of peace or concordance. Harmony is the main way in which feelings are expressed in music. Certainly, also used are lyrics, rhythm, tempo, and instrumentation. But in the musical texture, the horizontal expressions are melody and the vertical elements are chordal and harmonic progressions.

Dissonance within a chord produces tension whereas consonant chords produce release and rest. The dissonance within the chord creates the need for resolution, just as specific intervals, like the major seventh, yearn for resolution. Throw a seventh into a chord and you have interest and aural expectation. To recognize that a chord by itself does not have the immense impact it does without the harmonic placement and movement in the chordal progression is to know why score writers for movies are critical for the emotional impact of a movie film. What would *Star Wars* or *Gladiator* have been without the rich, full harmonic interest of either film score?

Minor harmonies sound sadder and major harmonies are brighter and more joyful. We use music and harmony to plumb the depths of ourselves as we listen to great music. Our composers reveal the most tender parts of a nation's soul through the harmony of her music. The harmonies that emerge in the music of a country paint the spirit and heart of her people. To know a culture, listen to her music. Her sacred core can be heard.

Instrumental and Vocal Timbre

Let us take a more in-depth look at the connection between the overtone series and *timbre*—the tonal quality of an instrument or voice that is determined by the overtones which are emphasized. Many variables are present to determine overtone array, and thus, the timbre of a sound. The size, material composition, and shape of an instrument contribute to the timbre. In voices, timbre is created by the resonant spaces in the mouth, throat, and torso, as well as by airflow and the general health of the individual.

Have you ever wondered why you can tell the difference between the voices of your friends? Or the difference between the sound of a flute and a trumpet even though both are playing the same pitch? It is because each sound has a different array of overtones or partial tones, heard and unheard pitches webbed into each unique sound. Some of the overtones are heard and some are not heard, but all contribute to the timbre, or unique sound, of the instrument or voice.

Overtones are present whenever a sound is made. The waves of sound have layers. Each layer vibrates at a frequency that is a multiple of the fundamental tone, which is the slowest wave and lowest tone—aka the pitch of the sound. A harmonic series is all the layers of frequency associated with the sine wave of the sound. A *partial tone* is any of the multiples that are present. These are all faster waves with shorter periods between their crests—so they sound higher.

Many times, overtones are folded into the perceived sound with the root pitch being the most dominant. As a voice teacher, I have trained myself to hear the very subtle overtones present in the voice of a students. Because sound requires a partially enclosed cavity to resonate, like the mouth, throat, or chest cavity, I can hear when the voice is not expressing its full capacity. If there is tightness in the body, the overtones will be dampened. That is why you can hear sadness or fear in a person's voice. Some of the perception of the voice is due to volume, but for the most part, it is tension present in the body that is producing the sound.

You can explore the harmonic series for yourself using your own voice by singing a fundamental note and altering the physical space in your mouth and throat. I have learned to produce this overtone series using my own voice, so it is clear to me that these pitch intervals are anchored into us in a visceral way.

Begin by sounding the vowel Ah on a comfortable pitch. Then slowly change the AH to an EE vowel and move to OO. Allow your tongue to move back and forth in your mouth on the OO vowel slowly changing the resonant space. The overtones will reveal themselves. You will continue to hear the fundamental pitch and the overtones will dance above that note.

We can create overtones easily, so perhaps they offer us a path, as if they were a clue for us to discover and follow.

As a voice teacher, I can hear where my student's tension is by recognizing which part of the body is closed simply by hearing the sound. For example, a voice that is produced by a person with a very tight throat has a very characteristic sound (imagine Kermit the Frog). The sound from a person with a tight and marginally opened mouth will also have specific sound (imagine Willy Nelson). From a healer's perspective, the parts of the body that are shut down can be addressed and opened to allow the production of a voice that is richer in overtones, and thus, more pleasing.

Is it any wonder that the voices of the great singers, such as Luciano Pavarotti, are beloved by so many? His voice was unique in the production of luminous overtones and could bring me to tears. It was as if the sound was a bridge to the realms of the divine. Coupled with the intention of love, it was rare that a person was not moved emotionally when listening to his glorious voice. I could hear love in his sound.

Which brings me to that inexpressible and mysterious quality that is heard in some voices: the sound of love. From research at the HeartMath Institute, we now know that the energies of love and compassion have a very high frequency, which can be measured within the electromagnetic field of the physical body.[1] Because of this, we know that if a voice carries these higher frequencies we are being bathed in love. Many instruments, such as gongs and crystal singing bowls, also are rich in higher overtones, and thus, may be used for sound healing.

The most healing energy we can feel, accept, and produce is love.

The Voice as an Instrument

What is the magic "it" that we hear in the voices of singers and speakers that draws us to them? We don't know yet, but we love the sound, want to listen to them over and over, feel better after listening to them, and are drawn into a "sound space" with them. I feel that this magic is sometimes just a gift, but that it also can be learned. It is the balance of body, mind, soul, and intention within the singer as the sound of his or her voice is released.

We are instruments of vibrational communication and our voices are the most powerful of the devices we possess. Our voices create resonance patterns within the environment near us and within the body. This can happen in a powerful and profound way when we are harmonically and energetically balanced and aligned. Our voice sends out a signal of the sum total of who we are into the vibrational field around us. As the fundamental resonance field of our body becomes free, clear, and healthy, our voice will mirror this positive condition and the field around us will carry the energy of vitality, health, and joy. This is the magic "it" that we hear.

If we are sick, depressed, wounded, or anxious, our voices will mirror these conditions as well. As singers and sounders and speakers, we have a power and sacred duty to contribute to our world in a positive and constructive way with voices that carry the highest ideals and most positive emotions possible. The body's mirror is very clearly and without a doubt, the voice.

This information is built on a comprehensive systemic view of the singer/speaker as a resonant instrument. To fully understand the phenomenon of the voice mirroring our internal condition (emotional and physical), let us review the basic knowledge of sound physics that demonstrates that as human beings, we are vibrational frequency fields. It is now clearly stated and acknowledged that at the quantum level, all matter is vibration, existing as either a wave or a particle at any given time, or more clearly, as either pure energy or matter. All matter has underlying energy. This knowledge is basic to the goal to be as resonant and responsive an instrument as is possible. All singers and speakers and sound healers must take the clarity and energetic health of their own bodies very seriously. Without a clear, open channel, the healing energy in sound, both spoken and sung, cannot easily flow.

Our bodies and souls are truly a harmonious, webbed interaction of vibrational energy. The balance and vitality of each of these aspects within the living system is a goal for every speaker/singer. In acoustical-patterning terms, health is the state in which the resonance of each body part (or component of the system)—thoughts included—is aligned with the resonance of all the other parts. When all parts are functioning harmonically together, we are literally "in tune" with ourselves. Attuned. It is as if all the instruments in a well-tuned orchestra were playing in the same musical key. A majestic synergy occurs and the whole becomes much more than the sum of the parts.

All matter can be viewed as patterns of vibration, so it can, in theory, be thought of as creating sound. The fields of sound that we hear are easy to identify however we are also moving through unheard fields of sound vibration around us. Nonetheless, they are unmistakably felt—levels of sound within our constantly vibrating world. Our world and all her inhabitants are "singing" together as a magnificent chorus of sound.

We literally can allow the cosmos to sing or speak through us. *Entrainment* is central to this phenomenon. Entrainment is the automatic synchronization of two vibrating objects that have the same natural frequency. A good example of this is when two tuning forks, made of the same material and tuned to the same frequency (for example, if both produce A tones) are placed next to each other and only one is struck. Because of entrainment, the second unstruck tuning fork will begin to sound the same note, influenced by the other.

As a further way to demonstrate this, I have also had my students sing into a piano while I hold down the damper pedal (which frees the strings to vibrate), and the string that matches the sung note will begin to sound. This is a very clear example of entrainment that is easy to experience.

Also, if a singer sings a note that matches one of the six guitar strings, the string matching the sung pitch will resonate. The sung note must be in the same octave of the guitar string.

If we can do entrainment with instrument strings and tuning forks, why could we not do it with people around us? Amazingly, we do this ALL the time with people around us. They resonate to our sound, and we to theirs. We become great and very effective healers when we resonate joy and compassion by inviting all within the energetic field to come into alignment with us by way of entrainment.

Thought is also vibration. We know that more positive thoughts vibrate at a higher frequency than heavier ones. The more positive energies, such as love, generosity, and compassion, have been shown through the work of Masaru Emoto to create more intricate and ordered patterns in frozen water crystals. He took pictures of frozen water crystals made from water that had been held in glass jars with words like *love* and *compassion* taped to the side of them. The resultant patterns were exquisitely beautiful. In contrast, water exposed to negative thoughts produced disordered crystals.

To remind you, our bodies are 80 percent water. If beautiful thoughts can create the ordered patterns in water crystals taken from lakes and streams, the same will happen in our bodies. Conversely, thoughts such as anger and aggression are likely to produce disordered patterns in the tissues of our bodies. These patterns could make us less able to produce resonant sound and energy fields.

Different thoughts, when generated by an individual, become integrated in the matrix of frequencies that individual is expressing and either encourage flow and dynamic motions of energy (both inside and outside the individual's body) or eventually manifest as disease, muscular tension, and energetic constriction. Emotional or physical trauma and despair create a dampening effect and cause energy to get stuck or become clouded and flow-resistant. Negative thoughts carry a powerful negative frequency that causes cellular structures to collapse.

The fastest way to shut down your voice is to carry anger, bitterness, resentment, or hostility in your heart. All of these states can be heard in the sound of the spoken and sung voice. A fully resonant voice cannot be produced if energetic resistance and/or physical tension is present.

Blocks to a Full, Resonant Voice

Psychological trauma sometimes causes past events to be stored in the energetic field of the body. The memory of an event is sometimes so traumatic that it bypasses the speech center and is processed by the limbic system in the brain which stores it as feelings and sensations. At the time of the event, the brain is so flooded with stress chemicals that processing the event is downshifted from the area of the neocortex (reasoning part of the brain) to the limbic system (the feeling part of our brain). Cognitive processes are not present at the time of the trauma as the person is drenched in survival modalities. Consequently, such an event lies in fragments, submerged in the psyche and stored in the body, which is unreachable through spoken language alone. Very often fragmented trauma is evident in a person's posture, manner of breathing, quality of the resonance in the spoken voice, quality of eye contact, and the rhythm of speech.

We know that energy, by way of the breath, can be withheld, released in spurts, or dampened. As singers and speakers, choosing when and how to release breath is fundamental to our art. We must have full and free access to our breath and energy.

As sound and voice healers, we can help people by calling the traumatic event into the consciousness using deep breath and sound. An event that has been stored in the body's tissues can be moved to the prefrontal cortex (thinking brain to be assessed, reordered, and finally integrated by the cognitive processes. In some cases, it is not even necessary to remember an event, it still must be given a voice to express its energy.

Crying, screaming, and moaning is giving voice to our response to a traumatic event. If these vocal reactions are suppressed at the time of an event, the entire body and vocal production suffer from the restriction and will compromise the release of energy, sound, and resonance. That's why people get shaky voices when describing upsetting events—even those from long ago.

The wholeness of a person's soul can be heard in his or her voice. A singer or speaker is not fully authentic or whole, until all of life's experiences have been integrated into the personality, brought into full awareness, and released from the unconscious. Unless unconscious trauma is processed, it will continue to restrict the voice and also to cry for attention by acting out in sabotaging behavior, phobias, and personality disorders. Everything must be brought out of the shadows and face the light of unconditional love.

I have been through this process and although it was painful, the alternative was unbearable. To live in shadow, covered by the darkness of my own unconscious pain was not full living. It was simply, coping.

We are not ushered into this mystical and magical experience called life to cope. We are here to evolve, flourish, and emerge as the magnificent beings that we were meant to be. The seeds of this deep knowing lie within each of us, waiting for us to turn to the knowing. No one, no person, no soul is left behind.

The greatest and most profound question we as a species can ask is "Who am I?"

I offer you an answer: love.

Forms of Musical Pieces and Sacred Music

In discussing the many forms of music, let us begin with the most common forms.

Strophic form is a repeated melody (AAA).

Binary form is a melodic line followed by a different melodic line (AB).

Popular song form or *ballad form* is fairly well known to us. The melody is introduced, thematically developed, and then a totally different melody, known as the *bridge* is introduced, and finally, we return to the original melody (AABA). Most popular music from the 1940s through the 1970s followed this melodic and harmonic structure.

Church hymns can be in strophic form, but many follow the verse and chorus form with the repeated chorus sung between different verses.

Gregorian chant could be considered *through-composed,* as most Gregorian chants (with the exception of Hildegard von Bingen's chants) did not repeat any melodic pattern. The melodic line continues to evolve with new melodic material.

A great deal of new age music is *through-composed,* as are the compositions that Daniel Wyman and I compose together. The result of through-composed music is the presentation of a flowing texture of consistently new melodic material and harmonic texture. Psychologically, the brain is not expecting to hear a melody repeated, and thus, it can relax in the flow.

Intention Behind Sound and Music

The energy or feeling in music is specifically connected to the quality of consciousness of the composer and the performer of that music. During my career as a classical opera singer I could "feel" when I had connected to the intention of the composer as I was performing the music. Crazy as it seems, there were times when I asked the spirits of Mozart and Bach to help me interpret a particularly difficult passage in a composition and the method and answer has appeared in a feeling.

Anytime I sing music of a different culture than my own, I learn as much as I can about it and then attempt to honor composer and culture by channeling the genuine feeling of the music. A Puccini aria has a different feeling than a Bach aria. A popular contemporary Mexican song is vastly different than a German art song that was composed in the nineteenth century.

Composers, whether from the same or different cultures, display different intentions and feelings. The music of Gabriel Fauré, for instance, has a quality that is heavenly and wondrous. His music can take my soul to places of radiance. The music of Mozart can be full of humor and joy. The music of each composer contains the heart and soul of that composer. It is an energy that is there to be expressed by a musician who recognizes that the process of singing or playing it is sacred and intensely intimate.

The deeper musicians have delved into their own souls, the more capable they are to join the soul expressions of a composer. Wrapped within every form of glorious music is gratitude, compassion, love, and a direct connection to Spirit. When we are in flow, we are merging and expressing Source . . . and we become . . . that.

The Power of the Heart in Healing

The HeartMath Institute (HMI) located in Boulder Creek, California, has contributed incredible new discoveries to us on the power of the heart in healing. Their research has found that when measuring the electromagnetic fields of the brain and the heart, the field of the heart is usually much larger. In his book *The Energetic Heart,* Rollin McCraty, Ph.D., states: "The heart generates the largest electromagnetic field in the body. The electrical field as measured in an electrocardiogram (ECG) is about sixty times greater in amplitude than the brainwaves recorded in an electroencephalogram (EEG)."[2]

HMI has also conducted studies to measure the power of intentional thoughts and emotions on human DNA. In a 2003 study, "Modulation of DNA Conformation by Heart-Focused Intention," Dr. McCarty and his colleagues Mike Atkinson and Dana Tomasino describe their experiment which proved this direct influence.[3] For the study, participants called *pilots* were asked to direct intentional, heart-centered, loving thoughts and intentions to samples of genetic material that they were holding in containers. The pilot was able to unwind the DNA double-helix spiral, which is a necessary precursor to replication, thus altering the confirmation of the cell's DNA.[4] For DNA to replicate, it must first unwind its spiral, break the ladder form in half, and allow RNA to replicate what it needs to complete the copy of the DNA.

Doc Childre, founder of HMI, has postulated that "an energetic connection or coupling of information" took place between the pilots' spirits and the DNA in cells.[5] Simply put, when an individual is in a state of loving compassion there is a direct flow from the divine expression of that individual to another person which can influence the systems, cellular structure, and health of the second person. He also has said: "Individuals who are able to maintain states of heart coherence have increased coupling to the higher dimensional structure and would thus be more able to produce changes in the DNA."[6] Coherence is defined as connection or consistency within the system.

Before I go on to explain how this information relates to music, I'd like to tell you about one more recent study, also directed by HMI, which is stunning in its results. The study, "Modulation of DNA by Coherent Heart Frequencies," conducted by Glen Rein, Ph.D., and Dr. McCraty, demonstrates that DNA is healed by harmonic entrainment with a compassionate heart.[7] The purpose was to test the impact of placing compassionate attention on DNA under controlled conditions. Dr. Rein coached pilots in biofeedback control by placing electrodes on their chests, thus training these individuals to create magnetic field coherence.

When the pilots were sufficiently skillful in creating heart-brain coherence Dr. Rein had them hold contained samples DNA mortally wounded by exposure to excessive heat. The pilots held these samples for an hour while focusing intentionally on compassionate love or universal love. Healthy DNA is formed by two long strands of protein that spiral to create the structure of the double helix. The chemical bases (ATCG) on one strand pair with the bases on another strand. Wounded DNA has connecting bases missing or damaged or the protein strand is damaged.

After the hour, Rein took a reading. In many cases, the DNA showed that the protein strands had healed; the bases had reconnected, and the double-helix form was present.

It is interesting to note that the structure of the DNA double helix shares the same golden ratio symmetry as the waveform of the piezo/sonic magnetic coherence that is produced by a heart which is focused on compassionate love. The golden ratio is sometimes referred to as a sacred geometry because it shows up in so many places in nature. The simplicity of this is at the core of my beliefs.

The conclusion of the study? Love heals.

As sound makers—and we are all sound makers by definition of being vibratory beings—we can offer healing energy to others by expressing love and compassion when we perform or speak, or when we are simply present. Our presence is a note played in the field of subtle energy. To be a healer may seem like an obvious choice, but the reality of life can lead us to put this noble intention and energy in suspension.

To be a portal for divine and loving energy, we must first face the shadows within us, and integrate all the attendant wisdom from all the experiences of our lives so that we may be fully authentic in our modes of self-expression and become carrier waves of compassion. We must offer both to ourselves without reservation or condition. When the divine, loving soul is fully anchored in the personality, and is its dominant driving force, the action of intention is very powerful. It is then as if we are using all the manifesting power of the divine field to bring into elegant display that which we have envisioned.

A wise person once told me words to this effect, and I paraphrase: "As you become more aware and awake to the divine essence that you are, you will manifest so quickly that it will make your head spin." I understand this remark now. A vision or dream fueled by love and joy is already on the horizon of your future experience.

Sacred Ritual

Sacred ritual is the container for intention. Our species has created ritual for millennia. Evidence of ritual practices reaches back 40,000 years into prehistory. Ritual signals safety and stability. It is any "religious or solemn ceremony consisting of a series of actions performed according to a prescribed order."[8] Without intention, however, a ritual is like a boat without a rudder adrift on the sea.

Because we know that what we envision using imagination has power and energy, to couple this with a divine purpose is deeply meaningful to us when we participate in a ritual. The ritual offers us a structure or container for a transcendent experience in which we literally enter another space and state of being which is separate from our daily lives.

The rituals that I experienced in Peru with the Shipibo Indians were powerful for me in that I felt a distinct energy descend into the ritual place, their maloca. It was clear to all taking part in any given ritual that this place at this time was unique and would be impactful. The rituals we did there readied my mind and spirit for deeper experience.

A ritual can be as simple as lighting a candle before meditation or saying words of gratitude before a family meal. It is a way to contain an experience in love.

Music can be the aural container for ritual in that it connects the heart to the sacred experience in a way that goes beyond the analytical mind. One is able to enter the spiritual space through the bridge of sound and music.

····································

FOUR

PSYCHOACOUSTIC ELEMENTS IN HEALING MUSIC AND SOUND

Sound resonances, and music, in particular, have a variety of psychological and physical effects on us that are good for our wellbeing.

Vibroacoustic Effects of Sound on the Human Biofield

The word *biofield* was designated by the National Institutes of Health in 1994 to describe the energy that surrounds the human body.[1] Each biofield is filled with information related to the emotions and experiences of the physical body which it encompasses and interpenetrates. Technology that is sensitive to electromagnetic energy (chi) can measure its characteristics. In the article "An Overview of Biofield Devices," David Muehsam, Ph.D., and Gaetan Chevalier, Ph.D., state:

Advances in biophysics, biology, functional genomics, neuroscience, psychology, psychoneuroimmunology, and other fields suggest the existence of a subtle system of "biofield" interactions that organize biological processes from the subatomic, atomic, molecular, cellular, and organismic to the interpersonal and cosmic levels. Biofield interactions may bring about regulation of biochemical, cellular, and neurological processes through means related to electromagnetism, quantum fields, and perhaps other means of modulating biological activity and information flow. The biofield paradigm, in contrast to a reductionist, chemistry-centered viewpoint, emphasizes the informational content of biological processes; biofield interactions are thought to operate in part via low-energy or "subtle" processes such as weak, nonthermal electromagnetic fields (EMFs) or processes potentially related to consciousness and nonlocality.[2]

A technology I am familiar with and use myself is a *gas discharge visualization* (GDV) technology. This device does electrophonic imaging; meaning, it collects electromagnetic information through the fingerprints (the hands are placed on metal plates) and correlates data with a catalogue of diagnostic information from the Chinese acupuncture system. The relative health of a subject is assessed through this technique, after which appropriate steps can be taken to restore the subject's body to healthy homeostasis. Collecting and assessing data about someone's electromagnetic health is key to employing sound and music as a curative modality.

Much of what we previously knew about the health benefits of sound and music came from the evidence of lowered blood pressure, reduced cortisol levels, and increase in immunoglobulin A and G levels, substances that signal an improved immune response. All these measures have demonstrated the validity of sound therapy.

Having newer technology, like the GDV device, that is able to assess the subtler energetic systems within the body is encouraging, as the body is far more than its material parts, like the bones, muscles, chemicals, and fluids. The body most certainly includes its subtle energy field.

The human energy field (biofield) or aura has been described in spiritual writing throughout recorded history, most notably in Buddhist and Hindu scriptures and medical texts from India and China. In the West, the symbolism of light associated with the body is found in the New Testament of the Christian Bible. In the King James version of the Bible, Matthew 6:22 reads:

> The light of the body is the eye. If therefore thine eye be single, thy whole body shall be full of light.

I find this remark fascinating as the pineal gland, which is located deep within the brain, often is referred to as the *third eye*. This gland has rods and cones within it, as do our eyes, and it is connected to the visual cortex of our brain. Is this what the biblical disciple Matthew was referring to in his description? And does the pineal gland help us to perceive subtle (nonphysical) information from the biofields around us? In my experience, it is possible for most people to see auras with some practice and guidance.

As described before, I believed my experience on the Connecticut Turnpike after my uncle's funeral opened this light-perceiving energy center in my head. Perhaps the intense love I was feeling allowed my pineal gland to be stimulated to a point that I had visions of light which seemed to be coming from outside my body.

Although the intensity of a body of light around the physical can vary—and in fact, biofields fluctuate all the time according to what's going on internally and externally—the way many people have described as the experience of observing auras sounds a lot like Matthew's description. Medieval paintings of spiritual nature also depict holy people with radiant halos around their heads which resemble emanations of light from the crown chakra.

Another word for the subtle energy of the aura is *bioplasma,* as is acts like an electromagnetic fluid surrounding the physical body. Like a fluid, it can vary in density and be observed has having lighter and darker variations. Typically, a normal body aura extends from the body at a distance of roughly five feet, certainly changing as emotions and intentions vary. When I sing in an auditorium for a large audience, as is the case with appearances with orchestras, I can sense my aura reaching the back walls of the auditorium. The biofield holding my intention of connection is riding on the sound of my voice, making it possible for me to have a direct interaction with every person in the audience. I know that it is possible to immediately change the energy in a room by the sound of a human voice.

Let us not forget the mesmerizing effect that Adolph Hitler had on thousands of Germans listening to him as he readied his country to go to war. The voice can be used to manipulate and control as well as to heal. A healing contrast to hostile charisma is the love I heard in Archbishop Desmond Tutu's voice as he spoke to the suffering population of South Africa during the era of the anti-apartheid and human rights movement. To this day, when I see a picture of him, my heart opens.

I believe we respond emotionally to all energy—even the energy we don't see but sense. If it was possible for me to see Tutu's aura from a distance, I am certain that it would encompass the world in compassion. It is possible. Love is without limits.

In the exploration of emotional imprints within our bodies of light, all our life experiences appear to be stored within this electromagnetic medium. The different stored emotions, as a result of experiences, have different frequency signatures. For example, fear has a very thick quality to it, whereas love possesses the qualities of lightness and softness. Other emotions, such as guilt, grief, and anger, have frequency signatures as well.

Imprints of emotions in an individual's biofield can come from various lifetime events that a person has experienced. When a traumatic event occurs, we do not evaluate the event analytically. The event is immediately stored in the limbic system, which is a gatekeeper for emotions stored within the brain. The imprint has a life of its own and is moved into the subconscious mind where it can become shadow. The more traumatic the event, the deeper the memory is hidden in the subconscious. Because we cannot access the subconscious mind (by definition it rides below our conscious awareness), the only way we can know what is there, is by our present-moment reactions to events. A clue that we have unprocessed memories (usually related to trauma) is if we react in the same way we did when the initial event impacted us.

For example, if someone speaks angrily to us and we fly into a rage it could be that our childhood home was full of conflict and we felt victimized by more powerful figures. We could not express the rage then, as we were children. So, we submerged the feelings about the events—and sometimes even memories of events—but we have a subconscious imprint that is triggered by harshness and anger. As an adult we may overcompensate for the past by overreacting in the present. These personal reactions may be a mystery to us until we understand the primal trigger, which was childhood abuse.

Although our imprints began as emotion felt in the physical body, they move into the energetic body and remain stuck there as negative and heavy energy. Many times, a disease will correspond with the location of one of these energy imprints, as imprints impede the free flow of life energy. In Traditional Chinese Medicine, a physician would say these spots have become stagnant.

Louise Hay in her seminal book, *You Can Heal Your Life*, describes the emotional cause of diseases. She draws a connection between negative thoughts and experiences and the diseases that are the results of these thoughts. I concur 100 percent with her assessments—which she intuited—as, over the years, I have interpreted all my own physical challenges through the lenses of my thoughts and experiences. Sometimes discovering a suppressed memory of a traumatic event is not a pleasant realization, but ultimately it is helpful and healing to bring it into the light and liberate the stagnant energy.

For example, I suffered with migraine headaches for years and tried every drug to both alleviate and avoid them. Many times, in the process causing myself more physical and emotional problems due to the side effects of the medications. Ultimately, I decided to heal myself as I was getting nowhere with drugs. Even so, the headaches persisted. Then I began to meditate daily to reconnect with a part of myself that was always at peace. I also changed my diet to avoid toxic and inflammatory foods and beverages.

The regimen took three years to return my body to a state of calm and health, but it worked. More recently, I added toning to my daily meditation and have noticed deeper, more consistent daily peace. My migraines now are gone. Without addressing the energetic cause, imprints can lead to chronic physical conditions.

In my quest to fully understand the source of my physical pain, I realized that the reason I initially suffered from migraines was my driving desire to achieve and be successful. I wanted to please my father, a very successful scientist who loved me but was not prone to demonstrate it. As an adult, I understood his inability, but there was still the child inside me who wanted her father's approval. Not that I blame him at all, as now I understand that it was my beliefs about his love that caused my distress. My beliefs created a painful emotional reality. He loved me deeply but not in a way a little girl could understand. I recognize now that I perceived things not as they were, but as I was, and so I had made a faulty decision that I was not loved just as I was.

In a way, the imprint has served me well, as I have achieved a tremendous amount thus far in my life. But there was a price to pay: The physical manifestation of the imprint was severe migraine pain. I finally freed myself by giving myself the approval I was seeking. My father can rest now. I love him, and I love myself. And the headaches are gone.

Sound can have a profound effect on subtle imprints even when we don't recall the cause of our initial trauma. Often crying accompanies the release of an imprint when we regain a lost memory, but the tears are welcome, as they are tears of healing. In the sound therapy sessions that I do with crystal singing bowls, many of my clients have reported that they don't know why they are crying. I explain that it is not necessary to know. We can trust that the release of pain and the return to a flow state is happening without a specific memory surfacing. A cathartic release indicates that the sound of the bowls has touched and activated an original traumatic energetic imprint, which is always either full of pain, fear, or sadness.

Certainly, the sound of crystal bowls has a marked effect on emotional and energetic imprints. Even more powerful is the effect of the sacred songs of the Shipibo shamans in the Amazon jungle. Before I made my own trip to Peru, a dear friend of mine recounted a journey to Peru she had made. She went deep into the jungle to stay at a sanctuary that offered her the opportunity to heal her ovarian cancer. This journey is not for the faint of heart, as the physical environment is difficult at best to traverse, but my friend was desperate. She felt that the cause of her disease was rooted in her destructive childhood relationship with her mother. She knew unprocessed and unresolved feelings had "gone underground" and suspected that the imprints of these were manifesting as cancer in her uterus.

Whether this was or was not so is not the point. SHE believed it, and thus, she left behind her definition of herself as a victim and became an activist in her own healing journey. She stayed in the Amazon for about a year working with a shaman and plant medicine. During this period, the hallucinogenic properties of ayahuasca and the powerful songs sung by the shaman enabled her to view the entirety of her subconscious and come to an understanding of the process of forgiveness and ultimately gratitude for ALL experience, including what had happened between her and her mother. She recounted that the icaros were like a surgeon's knife, as they sonically probed into her body and energetically cut out the imprint. My friend left the Amazon entirely cured and soon after became pregnant with a daughter, who is a wondrous being—now in her teens. This is truly a miracle story. And I have heard it repeated time and time again within the realm of love that is created by ayahuasca and the magic of the shaman's icaros.

After hearing about my friend's mystical journey, I resolved to experience ayahuasca myself, leading to the story I told you in Chapter 2 about my visit to the Shipibo sanctuary. To say that this was the most profound experience of my life to date is an understatement. Previously, I described the shamans' ceremonial process. Now I will explain more about how the sounds of the icaros sung by the shaman who worked with me interacted with the emotional imprints of suppressed trauma in my biofield.

Plant medicine takes about thirty minutes to begin to interact with the neurochemicals in the brain, which acts like a gatekeeper to a world of visionary experiences. The experience is known as a journey. Once that door is opened, colors and shapes descend on the "traveler" like a magnificent star shower. One can get lost in the beauty, but there are more gifts waiting as the ayahuasca penetrates deeper into the subconscious coaxing it to reveal its secrets.

The method of contacting such deep memories was achieved by the icaros. The shaman begins to sing these songs when they become aware that a healing process is underway. It is evident that there is an unnamable connection between the songs sung by a shaman, the biochemical action of ayahuasca within the body, and the unveiling of suppressed memories to the conscious mind. During the experience, the memories are reevaluated and understood from a divine perspective. The imprints are healed.

People have asked me if I was frightened or concerned during this experience, and my answer is no. I went to the Amazon knowing that at my core I am a divine spark and that my inner essence is love. So, I was ready to see and face anything in my subconscious that was not love and transmute those distortions into light.

I got my wish! Ayahuasca first took me into experiences within my first two marriages. I looked at where I had failed and forgave myself not with just words but at an emotional depth that went beyond words. I saw the lessons inherent in those relationships and finally came to unending and total gratitude for each of my former husbands. Both men gave me such gifts and wisdom. The pain within those marriages moved out of my biofield with copious crying. And when the catharses were over, the pain was gone. I was totally free and resting in the arms of love.

During the subsequent ceremonies, Mother Aya also allowed me to see the effects of past-life experiences on me and to discern the impact and influences of events within my past lives and my present life. For example, I began to see a pattern in which I have always been an outspoken and fearless advocate for truth. And I have been killed for it, sometimes in highly unpleasant ways. But let me say that the memories of my past-life deaths were not memories of physical pain but of the emotional terror experienced during those deaths. Today, I dedicated my life to encouraging and supporting my students and clients in their self-discovery of competence and self-love. Singing, speaking truth, and creating music have been central in how I offer a path to wholeness of spirit. To stand fearlessly in your own truth, no matter what that is, is an action of great courage and a gift to this world. Death is merely a change of clothes, nothing more. The soul continues in its endless discovery though countless lifetimes. The constant companions guiding me through these memories were the icaros being sung by the shaman.

Resonance

The sound of the icaros interacts with the human biofield in ways we do not totally understand. Some of the power of these songs comes from in the intention of the singer. Some comes from the resonant frequencies produced by the voice of the singer. Other variables may be the meaning of the lyrics sung and the unexplained metaphysically reality that the plant medicine energy might travel on the sound current. I do know that resonance plays a big part in the impact of the icaros. Three types of resonance are typically used by sound healers. They are:

- Resonance in spaces, or acoustic resonance.
- Resonance in materials, as in crystal bowls.
- Resonance in the quantum world, created by thoughts, intentions, and emotions.

Let's look at each of these in turn now.

Acoustic Resonance

Resonance in spaces happens when the wavelength of a sound equals the distance between two parallel walls. We have all experienced the sound of our voices in a tiled bathroom with its hard, resonant walls. It is easy to recognize that the sound is amplified. As a singer, I am very aware of where I am asked to sing and the influence of the acoustic resonance of the space on the quality of my sound and also the possible need for amplification.

When I sing at an outdoor event, I have always used amplification, as the sound of my voice does not have the advantage of walls to amplify it. In a church or a room with a high ceiling, however, the acoustic resonance of the room is quite helpful. Hard surfaces help as the soundwaves enjoy bouncing off them.

When I sing in a new indoor performance space, I walk around the room searching for the "sweet spot," a place where my voice is in sympathetic resonance with the room. There is an arching quality to my voice when I find this place, which is pleasing to hear.

Additionally, there are resonant spaces inside the body of the singer that is important for the voice student or a professional speaker to understand. Partially enclosed spaces, such as the mouth, the soft palate, and the throat are great places for the singers/speakers to explore as they strive for rich and resonant sound.

You can try this yourself by singing a tone and slowly opening and closing your mouth as you continue sounding the same pitch. You will hear the sound respond to the opening space and take on more color created by the addition of overtones—and the opposite.

It has been reported that beautiful vocal sound made in cathedrals, temples, or tombs like the King's Chamber in the Great Pyramid of Egypt can assist a person in being transported into higher state of consciousness. I believe a portal or bridge can be created by sound whereby an individual can experience these altered realms. The effect is due to the resonance of the architectural structure, and also the building materials.

Resonance of Matter

Part of the picture of various resonance frequencies has to do with a sound maker's biological matter, such as his or her bones, tendons, muscles, blood, and organs. The easiest of these to sense in your own body is your heart resonance. If you sing a scale while placing your hand over your heart you can feel and hear the note that has the most power both in sound and in feeling. Try it now.

To chant or tone on this pitch can be a transformative experience, as you are stimulating the heart chakra and increasing its energetic presence. The chakras themselves are vortices that have resonant frequencies, or pitches, that are in sympathy with the organs that are under their influence. These pitches can vary among individuals, but most people would agree that the pitch of the root chakra, the lowest major chakra in the body, is the note C (Do). The other six chakras ascend from there, following the pitches of the diatonic scale: C, D, E, F, G, A, B.

The chakras will be discussed in depth in a later chapter. For now, it is prudent to note that the entire human body is an orchestra of resonant frequencies. Cells also have their own resonant frequencies, which can be picked up by extremely sensitive microphones. Michael Feld and Subra Suresh, researchers at the Massachusetts Institute of Technology, have measured the frequency at which red blood cells vibrate and shown that these frequencies reflect the health of the cells.[3] They were able to observe the vibrations of the membrane of a malaria-infected blood cell and then to correlate its changing vibrational frequencies during the progression of the disease. Apparently, every cell has electrical, chemical, and biological activity within its walls that causes nanoscale vibrations at its surface.[4]

Another cutting-edge researcher and musician mentioned earlier, Fabien Maman, conducted research in the early 1980s at the Jussieu Campus of the Pierre and Marie Curie University in Paris, France. He photographed the impact of sound on human cells and the attendant energy fields. He discovered that exposure to an ascending scale from C–D–E–F–G–A–B–C–D would explode cancer cells while leaving healthy cells unaffected.

After placing human uterine cancer cells on slides, Maman mounted a camera on a microscope to observe the effect of various instruments played for twenty minutes. "The structure quickly disorganized. Fourteen minutes was enough time to explode the cell when I used these nine different frequencies,"[5] says Maman, as he describes music killing cancer cells.

However, Maman found that the most dramatic influence on the cells came from subjecting the cells to the human voice as the cancer cells exploded within nine minutes. He says: "The human voice carries something in its vibration that makes it more powerful than any musical instrument: consciousness. It appeared that the cancer cells were not able to support a progressive accumulation of vibratory frequencies and were destroyed."[6] As I pondered why this would be the case, the example of an opera singer shattering a glass by singing a very high note came to mind. I have experienced this phenomenon when I shattered the glass in a picture frame by singing a high C. I believe that as the resonant frequency of the glass was exactly the frequency I was singing, it could not hold form when the note with all accompanying overtones was sounded. Perhaps this is the same action that Maman demonstrated with the cancer cells. He also reports finding that the frequencies of A at 440 Hz and B at 493 Hz caused the cancer cells to lose their structure and break down. The normal cells remained intact, however, and, in some cases, became stronger.[7]

In summary, there is solid science to back up claims made for the healing properties of vocal toning. The evidence goes far beyond the level of "it feels nice, so it must be good for me."

In 2000, I had the honor of attending one of Maman's workshops in the south of France under the auspices of the Academy of Sound, Color, and Movement he founded. I clearly recognized through my study that summer how color and movement are integral in the healing action of sound.

And so, we begin to see that specific resonances produce distinctive effects on energetic emotional imprints and also on diseases that invade the cells of the body, like cancer and viruses.

A scientist who was aware that cancer cells could be eradicated with a specific targeted frequency was Royal Rife (1888–1971), an American inventor. Rife believed that viruses were the cause of cancer, which at that time was a revolutionary concept. We now know that 16 percent of cancer is caused by viruses, such as the Epstein-Barr virus and the hepatitis B virus, among others. In the 1930s, Rife invented an optical microscope with which he could observe microbes that were too small to see with his era's available technology. Following this, he was able to discern the energetic frequencies needed to destroy cells damaged by many diseases. His research was suppressed and confiscated by the American Medical Association.[8]

Resonance in the Quantum Field

Hang on, dear reader, because we are about to jump down the rabbit hole by zooming into the quantum world to discuss resonance in this magnificent realm. Let me first declare that quantum fields do not interact with matter. Quantum fields ARE matter. In quantum field theory, what we perceive as particles are simply vibrations within the quantum field itself. Two fields exist, one within the other: the electromagnetic field and the electron field. As energy is created by the momentum of the push-pull of electromagnetism, the electrons are excited and created.

Quantum science is the study of the nature and behavior of matter and energy at both the atomic and subatomic level. This field of study, arising in the early part of the twentieth century, was a direct opposite of Newtonian physics, which describes the physical forces in nature that occur on a larger scale. Said another way, Sir Isaac Newton's laws of classical physics predict the relationship between a large body of matter, the forces acting upon it, and its motion in response to those forces. Newtonian classical physics can predict with certainty the trajectory of an apple dropping from a tree. Quantum physics is the physics of probabilities at the atomic and subatomic levels. If the apple was as small as a subatomic wave of energy, the trajectory of that "apple wave" could only be considered by probability.

For me, studying quantum physics was a call to enter the crazy and delightful world of *Alice in Wonderland*. Maybe all the spiritual knowledge I had studied and learned could be explained within the foundation of this emerging physics describing the subatomic world? Like many other nonscientists, I became fascinated with this world and the implications of quantum physics in the late 1980s when the advance of string theory became a hot topic.[9] As a vocalist and musician, I loved the vision of microscopic strings vibrating within matter, as with vibration always comes sound. Reports of this quantum phenomenon perked my ears up considerably. Then the older research in wave/particle duality flooded the meditation and metaphysical healing scene and I was sold. We know through these studies that energy waves change state when observed, going from waves to particles.[10] Consciousness and its connection to energy and matter was now being considered.

The new physics tells us that the difference between matter and energy is the state of vibration or speed of its oscillations. This knowledge, which has become mainstream for the quantum physics community, began with Thomas Young in 1801 demonstrating the wave function of light through a double slit. It was repeated in 1923 by Clinton Davisson and Lester Germer, demonstrating the diffraction patterns of electrons, and by Louis de Broglie in 1924, at last proving particle-wave duality.[11]

In essence, we now know that light can either express itself as a wave, which is energy, or a particle, which is matter. Subsequent research done by theoretical physicist David Bohm has shown that the deciding factor for either of these two expressions occurring under laboratory conditions is the directed attention (or consciousness) of the observer. Bohm's theory has enormous implications for us, as we live in a world of both particles (matter) and waves (energy/information/frequency). Let us try to make sense of our qualitatively dual reality and see how the discovery applies to sound, healing, and our daily lives. Sound and music, because of their vibratory nature, help us to explore this vast new world of the field of seen and unseen energy, which in Albert Einstein's terms, was everything.[12] If we look at our surroundings with fresh, unbiased eyes, we might be able to see that everything, including our bodies, the chairs, the buildings, is simply energy formed into different shapes. A chair is energy that has "collapsed" (Bohm's term) into formed matter.

To continue to explore this *Alice in Wonderland* world of quantum "magic," let us consider the atom. We know that the atom is mostly space and that atoms are the building blocks of matter. Let me give you an idea of the amount of space in an atom. All atoms have a core, called a *nucleus*, which is encircled by different numbers of *electrons,* that act like orbiting satellites. If the nucleus of an atom were the size of an orange, the electrons that circle the nucleus would be circling it at the distance of the circumference of the Earth. The rest of the atom is SPACE. But that space is not devoid of content, just matter. It is full of wave energy, which is saturated with information, just like the radio waves in a room are full of information.

We would need a very special radio to decipher the energy in an individual atom, but it is there nonetheless. It really is the same with the space in a room. There is infinite information present.

I will take this description a step further. Albert Einstein stated that everything is in motion.[13] If so, I posit that everything creates sound because everything is vibrating. Known or not, we are saturated with, and are swimming in sounds.

Physicist Nassim Haramein, founder of the Resonance Science Foundation in Kilauea, Hawaii, has discovered the energetic geometric shape of 99.999 percent of space at the quantum level. Knowing that sound creates shape in matter (cymatics), he noted that there seemed to be a correlation between sound and shape and to uniquely specific shapes often referred to as *sacred geometry* (geometry that is repeatedly displayed in the physical world, such as the shape of the spiral). His groundbreaking research, which is shaking up the scientific community, has led to the further exploration of the geometric template for all matter at the quantum level, which is the star tetrahedron.[14]

In Figure 4.1, on the next page, we can see the star tetrahedron, which has appeared in the art of world cultures throughout history. From Spain and Greece, to China and the Middle East, different cultures have drawn two-dimensional representations of this shape. Why? *Why has this shape been seen in art from antiquity to the present day?* This was a question that I pondered for many months.

The most fundamental quality of the star tetrahedron is that it is a geometry of absolute equilibrium and, therefore, great stability. It is, in theory, the geometry of the vacuum of

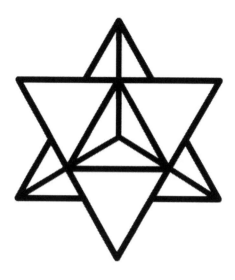

Figure 4.1: The star tetrahedron.

space, emblematic of the zero-point energy within the unified field. For anything in the universe to be manifested, either physically (as would occur in energy and matter) or metaphysically (as would occur in a field of consciousness), it requires a fluctuation in the unified field. Zero-point energy is the lowest energy state possible in a quantum system.

Through the study of cymatics (full explanation in the following chapter) and appreciating that sound is the generating force that forms all of the geometric patterns seen throughout our natural world, I have drawn some conclusions. Foremost: Sound must be the initiator of all manifestation at the zero-point level. My speculation is that the star tetrahedron is the repository of the creative energy sitting in total equilibrium until sound generates an emerging form. No other geometric shape has folded within its boundaries all the geometric shapes known as *platonic solids*—the tetrahedron, the cube, the octahedron, the dodecahedron, and the icosahedron.

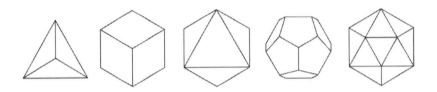

Figure 4.2. The platonic solids.

The platonic solids are shapes that reflect our three-dimensional world. I believe that sound generates the fluctuation in the unified field from which matter emerges in primal states. Because the star tetrahedron is a shape that holds dynamic possibilities within it, it constantly interacts with everything, receiving and storing information, swirling in a toroidal action from wave to particle and energy to matter, sound, and frequency. It can manipulate and constantly create new responses to the environment.

Our world of sound has a profound influence on us, physical, emotionally, and spiritually. We respond to sound and music because, at the basic quantum level, we are 99 percent space, information, possibility, vibration, and frequency in the form of waves and quantum particles. We are saturated with the sounds around us—and webbed into them. In fact, at the quantum level, everything is connected to everything else in a very real way. It's not metaphorical. We are the orchestra around us. We are the instruments, the musicians and the energetic field surrounding it all.

I can say without reservation that sound is the mother of us all.

Resonant Fields of Sound

A *sound field* is the technical name given to the presence of sound energy within given architectural boundaries, such as the walls, floor, and ceiling of a room. The space within a gothic cathedral is a marvelous example of architectural boundaries that produce strong and resonant sound fields. Once experienced, you will always remember the feeling of hearing music in such a space. It is necessary to be within the space to fully appreciate the effect. Hearing the recorded sound of choral singing in a gothic cathedral does not give the listener/experiencer the same feeling as being there in person. That is because recorded music is compressed.

Audio compression is the process of equalizing the dynamic range between the loudest and quietest parts of a recording. As equality is achieved, the audio signal is diminished. So, what a recording offers is not the same as the live sound, which has the loud and soft signals in full array. The physical experience is consequently dampened.

LIVE music is the most powerful and extraordinary physical experience for a true music lover. This awareness is important for those who would use music to heal. The creation of healing sound fields must be produced by live sound.

I remember an experience I had as a soloist for a production of Ludwig van Beethoven's Ninth Symphony. The forces needed to fully honor Beethoven's wishes are extraordinary. The orchestra numbers close to one hundred musicians and the size of the chorus is about the same. I was sitting in front of the orchestra waiting for the last movement of the symphony, which is when the soloists sing. The music was beyond glorious and as the time approached when I would stand up and sing, I found myself overcome with the emotion that only comes in the presence of profound beauty. To be immersed by the open hearts of over 200 people unified within this piece that is like a magnificent musical prayer, this love-filled sound, was overwhelming. I did sing the soprano solo parts and, as I remember, it was as if I myself was not singing, but that another force had moved into my body and produced the sound. I felt and experienced heaven that night in that resonant field of love.

The combined fields of all the people involved in making music on that occasion created an immensely powerful field that was much stronger than what would have been created by the separate fields of these people performing alone. The phenomenon of *resonance dominance* was also in play that night. This is the ability of one vibration to change another vibration. We feel this effect as we become entrained to a higher vibratory state by simply being in the presence of a positive person. The audience that came to the performance of the Ninth Symphony that evening may have come with frequency signatures of anxiety, depression, or sadness, but I would bet my life that they did not leave that way. It would have been impossible to hold the resonance of sadness within that powerful field of love. I have no way of proving this, of course, but it is my unshakeable belief.

The Overtone Series and Its Connection to the Major Triad

To clarify more deeply, the overtone series that we touched upon in Chapter 2 is a series of pitches that are enveloped within the totally perceived sound of an instrument or voice. A *sine wave sound* has no overtones as the only sound is the fundamental pitch. Before 1997 in the United States, we heard this sound at times when there was a TV or radio test of the Emergency Broadcast System interrupting our regular programming with a high-pitched whine. Since 1997, this capability is called the Emergency Alert System.

With any natural sound, overtones are heard in different gradations of loud to soft, and these give the sound its unique character. A clarinet, for example, has a different sound than a flute because you are not just hearing the fundamental pitch, you are also hearing countless notes in the background that are webbed into the fundamental pitch of the instrument. The relative strengths or weaknesses of those other pitches (called *overtones* or *partials*) give the instrument its characteristic sound.

When you hear the voice of a good friend, you can identify that person when your friend only says hello. That is because the signature sound of your friend's voice is created by the various overtones that are present. All tones are present, but some are louder than others when different people speak.

The overtones for each fundamental pitch follow a set pattern. For example, the fundamental note C has its first overtone an octave above the fundamental (another C). The second overtone is always a fifth above that, or a G. The third overtone is yet another C and lies a fourth above the second overtone. The fourth overtone is a third above the C and is an E, which completes our major triad in sound. The fifth overtone is again the fundamental pitch of C.

The overtone series explains a scientific fact. Whenever you strike a note on a piano or play one on a clarinet, you are not simply listening to that one note. There are countless other notes quietly humming about in different gradations of loud or soft, all of them below our threshold of conscious hearing. The relative strengths and weaknesses of these additional notes gives the sound its own particular character. This is why you would never mistake a clarinet for a piano.

Interestingly, these partials are all pitched higher than the note you actually played, and they vibrate at the same distance from that note and from each other in the case of all musical instruments. In other words, there is only one overtone series.

If you are familiar with the piano, the following illustration will make sense to you. Figure 5.3 shows the first sixteen overtones in order. This specific series is built on the fundamental note of C

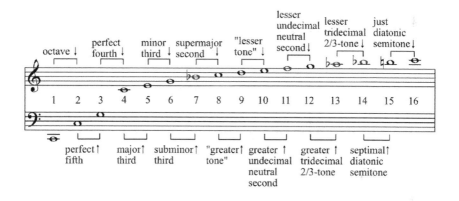

Figure 4.3. The overtone series in the key of C.

Within the overtone series, the fundamental pitch, C, takes center stage. It is expressed four times flanked by E and G, to form a *major triad*, from my perspective the most healing chord. These are the first three notes in the song "Kumbaya," a folksong whose origins are the Gullah-Geechee people of coastal Georgia and South Carolina, a melody popularized in the 1950s and 1960s.[15]

In *Harmonielehre* (German for *Theory of Harmony*, a book published in 1906, Heinrich Schenker calls a major triad the "chord of nature" and elevates it to an almost mystical presence.[16] He may be right about the connection to nature, as early Pythagorean students found that if a taut string was halved, the new pitch of one-half was an octave above the original string (C to C). If the C string was divided into thirds, the resultant pitch was a perfect fifth above the original (G).

If the C string was divided into four equal parts, again a C resulted—this time two octaves above the original. If the same original string was divided into five equal parts, an E pitch resulted. And lastly, if it was divided into six equal parts, we would arrive back to the fundamental pitch of C. So here again, our magnificent major triad gleams in its simplicity.

In further exploration of overtones, as I mentioned before, I learned how to produce them with my voice in much the same way that the Mongolian throat singers produce overtone above the fundamental pitch. They essentially are singing two pitches at once. Granted, the vocal folds are producing only one pitch, but by manipulating the resonant spaces in the mouth, it is possible to uncover the overtones folded within the sung pitch. So, my thought is that the major triad is enveloped and integrated into our bodies representing in aural terms, a balanced and flowing energetic system.

························

FIVE

THE ENERGY OF FREQUENCY, FORMS, AND BIOFIELDS

C ymatics, from the Greek word *kyma*, meaning "wave," is the study of sound vibration made visible.

Cymatics

Through sound vibrations influencing matter, we can see the transformational nature and direct correspondence of sound and matter. Sound surrounds, penetrates, and guides us, yet, until recently in human history, it has been an invisible force. Today we can see sound in audio waveforms but that is only a two-dimensional view. The magical world of cymatics, however, gives us a different view of both two- and three-dimensional representations of sound. This field of study, initiated by Hans Jenny in the 1970s, has offered us a major evolution in our understanding of how sound influences us.

Cymatics proves that everything that appears as matter, including the human body, is vibrating at its own rate. Cymatics merges the fields of sound and geometry into one, through the display of extraordinary images created by various sound frequencies. Typically, to produce an image the surface of a plate or membrane is vibrated by specific frequencies. Regions of maximum and minimum particle displacement become visible in the thin coating of sand or other particles lying on the plate or within liquid saturated with particulate that is situated on the plate.

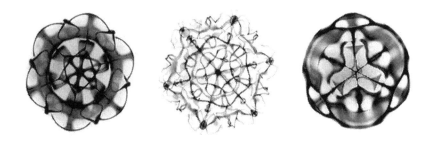

Figure 5.1. Cymatic patterns of sound made visible.

The extraordinary phenomena of cymatics were first noticed in the eighteenth century by Ernst Chladni, a German musician and physicist. Chladni allowed the physics of sound to be displayed by using a violin bow to vibrate a metal plate with sand on it to create geometric shapes. He discovered that the fine sand moves due to the vibration and accumulates in lines upon the surface of the plate. He called these *nodal lines of the vibration mode*.[1] If the parameters of the experiment were consistent, the result was repeatable. His work was foundational in the future development of cymatics. In 1787, Chladni published his findings in his book *Entdeckungen uber die Theorie des Klanges*, or *Discoveries on the Theory of Sound*.

In 1967, Hans Jenny repeated Chladni's experiments and drove the study of sound made visible into a new phase of deeper discovery. Jenny put sand, dust, and viscous fluids on metal plates connected to a frequency oscillator, which could produce a very wide spectrum of sound. He found that his materials organized into different structures driven by the frequency of the vibration coming from the oscillator or sound source.[2] These images are amazing, to say the least, as the natural forms and images in nature are revealed in these cymatic forms.

In the Bible, John 1:1 reads, "In the beginning was the Word, and the Word was with God, and the Word was God."[3] Similarly, the even more ancient Hindu scriptures read, "In the beginning was Brahman with whom was the Word, and the Word is Brahman."[4] Whether or not John had exposure to these texts we cannot know. But I appreciate that people for millennia have related to this sacred information, as it is also my belief that sound is the generating force for all of creation. All matter comes from the womb of divine sound.

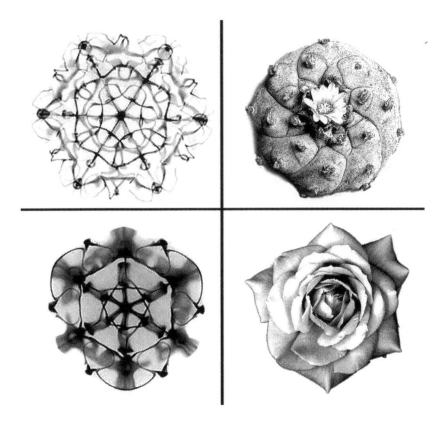

Figure 5.2. Forms from nature resemble cymatics-produced images. On the top right, across from a corresponding image, is a peyote button. On the lower right is a rose.

Sound eclipses the proverbial mystery "Which came first, the chicken or the egg?" in that primordial sound has created both.

Hans Jenny further posits that sound and its resultant patterns are a manifestation of an invisible forcefield of vibrational energy that spawns all of creation. He observed that when the ancient Sanskrit sound OM (thought to be the sound of creation by both Hindus and Buddhists) was vocalized over lycopodium powder, the shape that emerges is a circle with a center point in the middle of the circle. Since antiquity, OM has been represented in this way. The ancients must have understood cymatics.

Another leader in the world of cymatics is Alexander Lauterwasser, a photographer who has made images of cymatic patterns on the surface of water. Sound sources he has used include the sound of pure sine waves, vocal music, and orchestral compositions by Beethoven.

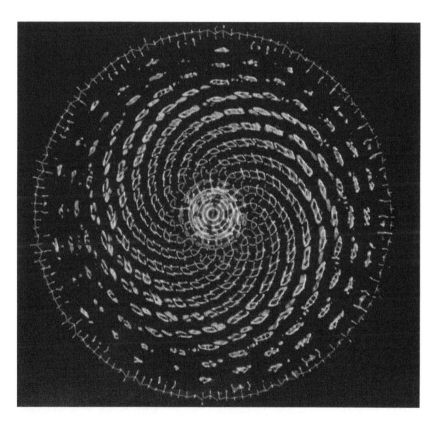

Figure 5.3. Lauterwasser images of sound patterns in water.

Simply by observing the patterns in Lauterwasser's photographs, we can begin to see these patterns as the seeds of creation of everything from galaxies to the human eye. The question arises: "Does the genesis of all matter flow from sound?"

Hans Jenny states:

The more one studies these things, the more one realizes that sound is the creative principle. It must be regarded as primordial. No single phenomenal category can be claimed as the aboriginal principle. We cannot say, in the beginning was number, or in the beginning was symmetry, etc. These are categorical properties which are implicit in what brings forth and what is brought forth. By using them in description we approach the heart of the matter. They are not themselves the creative power. This power is inherent in tone, in sound.[5]

When observing a frequency sweep imposed on sand sprinkled on a plate, the studies show that there is a moment when pattern chaos is present before the next tone is sounded. In other words, as the pitch rises and before the next tone is sounded, chaos rather than order is evident in the sand. What is happening is that the matter is rearranging itself into a new form based on exposure to a new frequency.[6]

This finding has truly great implications for us as beings of matter, as we also are subject to frequency sweeps in our natural environment. Chaos always strives for order in form. Perhaps this is why I love the peace and frequency stability of my ranch in the Hill Country of Texas. I can come home after a day in traffic and the sound pollution of town noise and feel myself respond to the healing frequency of Mother Earth and her critters, my horses and goats. I am once again aligned with that sound frequency of nature rather than the chaos of competing frequencies.

Truly, it is humbling to think that sound can create so much intricate beauty and peace. Geometry represented by cymatic images contains reoccurring themes, like spheres, hexagons, star tetrahedrons, and triangles. The implications of these emerging shapes will be discussed in the next section on sacred geometry, which is the geometry of the natural world.

As we begin to appreciate and connect with our natural environment, we are sure to notice the noise pollution of cities and the affects it can have on us. If one tone can create these imprints, imagine what unordered shapes related to harsh or unnatural sounds can have on our bodies. I believe that the vibrational geometry of nature can bring us back into balance while noise pollution and increasing electromagnetic fields around us drain our energy and cause disease.

The study of cymatics by Ernst Chladni and Hans Jenny began as visual experiments and now this research has evolved to encompass sacred geometry, metaphysics, philosophy, and the impact of our sonic environment on our wellbeing, which, of course, is an important foundation for the art of sound healing.

Sacred Geometry

As stated above, sacred geometry is the geometry of our natural world. It involves universal patterns that appear in the design of all reality. My belief is that there is a geometric and mathematical ratio infused into our natural world.

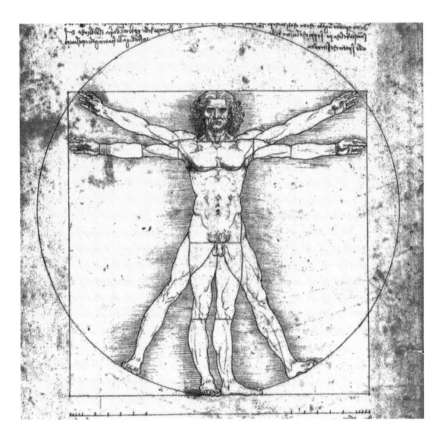

Figure 5.4. The Vitruvian Man, a drawing by Leonardo DaVinci, circa 1490 displaying balanced mathematical proportions and physical symmetry.

These ratios are also evident in music, proportions of living beings, and cosmology. The famous drawing "The Vitruvian

Man" (circa 1490) by Leonardo DaVinci is a perfect example of the sacred proportions expressed in the human form.

We see the same geometric proportions repeated in architecture, symbols, religious structures, and spaces that we find harmonious, leading to the impression of a grand design. The seed of life pattern also reflects this geometry.

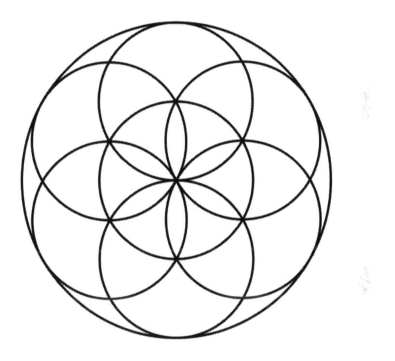

Figure 5.5. The seed of life pattern.

Other notable examples of the same sacred proportions are the chambered nautilus and its shell (see figure 5.6 on page 122), which form the shape known as the Fibonacci spiral.[7]

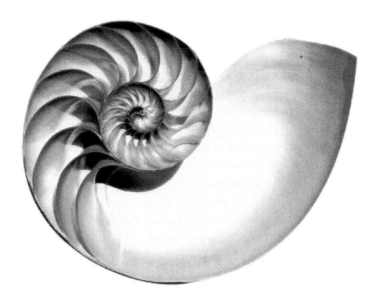

Figure 5.6. The chambered nautilus shell, which grows in the spiral shape endemic throughout the natural world.

There seem to be repeating patterns of great significance strewn before our eyes like clues awaiting discovery. The shape of the galaxies, hurricanes, the human eye, water spinning down a drain all display the same spiral. The proverbial "elephant in the room" is the question, Why? Why is this infinitely repeating pattern evident in all things?

My belief is that sound is the seed, the mother of all matter, and from the unified field of possibilities it brings into form all solid expressions from within the webbed geometry of the star tetrahedron in the unified field existing as waves of possibility and infinite potential.

We are truly beings of light, as is everything around us.

The Number 432 and 432 Hertz Tuning

Let me first say that there has been some confusion about the number 432 and 432 Hz. The number 432 has a great deal of mystical associations, which I shall address shortly. However, the PITCH of 432 Hz is an A.

Tuning to 432 Hertz

The pitch of A is what orchestras throughout the world tune to before a concert so that all the instruments match in frequency. When you hear the oboe begin the tuning process, the musician will sound out an A. The A that is used today is an A at 440 Hz rather than 432 Hz, which is just a bit lower in pitch. True, the difference is slight, but it can be perceived by the ear and has profound effects on our bodies. When we compare the cymatic representation of both of these pitches, side by side (see figure 5.7 on the next page), it is evident that the cymatic representation of 432 Hz is a much more well defined and intricate a pattern. Subjectively, it is felt and experienced as more pleasing.

Eric Rankin, screenwriter of the documentary *Sonic Geometry*, said that music and sound are mathematically consistent with the patterns of the universe when we tune our instruments to A at 432 Hz. Even so, the 440 Hz tuning has been the accepted universal tuning standard since the World War II era. Various conspiracy theorists have implicated the Nazi German war machine as the driving force

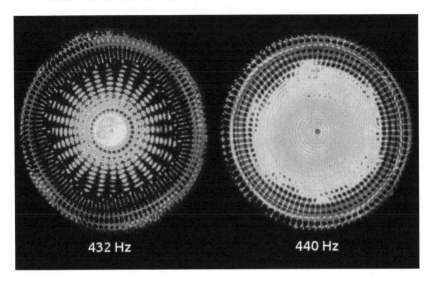

Figure 5.7. The waveforms of 432 Hz (left) and 440 Hz (right). This is an artist's interpretation based on photography of soundwaves in water.

behind this change in tuning practices. Ostensibly, the reason was to create feelings of unrest and dissatisfaction among the German people as they listened to music in the higher tuning.[8] Whether this is true or not, the higher tuning does create feelings of anxiety, whereas instruments tuned to A at 432 Hz make music that is more centering and calming to the listener. However, we cannot forget the research of Fabien Maman who notably used A440 to explode cancer cells.

The American Federation of Musicians accepted the A440 as standard pitch in 1917; however, it was not until 1959 that this pitch was accepted internationally. Before recent times, a variety of tunings were used, but A432 was very common in

France and in Italy before 1940. The composer Giuseppe Verdi was adamant about his opera orchestras tuning to A432 as he said that operatic voices singing with these orchestras were more powerful and more beautiful.[9] I am an opera singer and I can tell you that singing an aria from *La Traviata* accompanied by instruments tuned to A432 is much easier on the soprano voice than when the orchestral instruments are tuned to A440. I am sure that the explanation is that vocal music in 432 Hz is consistent with the sacred geometry and mathematical ratios present in our bodies. The sound and the body geometry are complementary.

I have listened to many examples of the same musical piece tuned to the different A pitches. Subjectively, I can feel the difference and energetically I relax more into the music if the instruments are tuned to A432 Hz. Because, I believe, the sound is consistent with my physical geometry. Seeing the Figure 5.7 images was proof enough to me to give my body and ear the more exquisite sound by listening to music in 432 Hz.

Sonic Geometry and the Number 432

Sonic geometry is a description of how sound frequency relates to form in the most exquisite and amazing way. Mentioned above, Eric Rankin, a new thought pioneer, and his colleague Alanna Luna concluded that there was a direct and stunning correlation between two-dimensional and three-dimensional geometry and sound frequency. They began asking the questions that ultimately uncovered the connection between geometrical shapes, and sound. The initial investigatory question was: What would happen if the sum of angles of all shapes were played as musical frequencies or pitches?[10]

What emerged from Rankin's and Luna's question was information that will forever influence how I view and value sound as an aid to healing—and ultimately, the ascension of the human spirit. He believes that hidden in the mathematical system based on the numbers 12 and 60 used by the early Bronze Age Sumerian culture (4000–1900 B.C.E.) is the enigmatic number 432. According to the Sumerians, this mysterious number was given to them by their sky gods, the Annunaki.[11]

Even today, 12 and 60 are endemic in how we measure and calculate time, distance (inches), and mathematically describe geometry. The number twelve is also evident in our numbering history. For example, in the twelve disciples of Jesus Christ, the twelve signs of the Zodiac, the twelve hours of day and of night, the twelve months of the year, and the list goes on and on.

The number 432, which is a multiple of 12, but not of 60, is recurrent in the ancient measurements of earth cycles, such as the Hindu timeline. The Kali Yuga (an age said to be ruled by the demon Kali, not the goddess Kali) lasts 432,000 years.[12] Four hundred and thirty-two is the only whole number that, when squared, comes within .01 percent accuracy of the speed of light, which is 186,624 miles per second.

Other examples of its appearance are:

- The number of seconds in a twenty-four-hour period are 86,400, and in a twelve-hour period 43,200.
- The diameter of the sun in miles (86,400), which is 200 times 432.
- The diameter of the moon is 2,160 miles, 432 multiplied by 5.

The number 432 was used as a measure in the construction of many ancient sacred sites, such as the Great Pyramid of Egypt. It is said that 432 Hz vibrates with the universe's golden mean Phi (the ratio, or proportion, 1.618...) and unifies the properties of light, time, space, matter, gravity and magnetism with biology, the DNA spiral and consciousness. More simply said, when our atoms and DNA start to resonate through sound and harmony with the toroidal spiraling patterns of nature, our sense of connection to nature is magnified. We are essentially reflecting the same pattern and toroidal spin present in all atoms when we are bathed in sound that is tuned to A432.

The F-Sharp (F#) Major Triad

A deeper exploration of 432 as it applies to frequencies emerges if a frequency tuning grid begins with A at 432 Hz. An astounding picture is created as we begin to build this grid with each note and frequency separated by 9 Hz. The number 9 and the number 432 have many commonalities. The number 9 is the sum of 4 + 3 + 2. We find that if we tune to A432 Hz and begin to represent each subsequent note by increasing or subtracting 9 Hz, it is revealed within the grid the sum of the angles of all two and three-dimensional shapes. All the notes are represented in the Hertz of whole numbers, not fractions. Additionally, all the individual numbers of the frequencies add up to 9.

"Factor 9" Grid Built on 432

C	126	252	504	1008	2016
C#	135	270	540	1080	2160
D	144	288	576	1152	2304
D#	153	306	612	1224	2448
E	162	324	648	1296	2592
F	171	342	684	1368	2736
F#	180	360	720	1440	2880
G	189	378	756	1512	3024
G#	198	396	792	1584	3168
Ab	207	414	828	1656	3312
A	216	432	864	1728	3456
A#	225	450	900	1800	3600
B	234	468	936	1872	3744
B#	243	486	972	1944	3888

Figure 5.8. The factor 9 grid. The shaded numbers correlate with various geometric shapes (see figure 5.9).

When we tune A to 440 Hz, the synchronicity fails. No sums of geometric angles are revealed in the 440 Hz grid and the notes must be represented by the addition of fractions.

As you can see in the factor 9 grid (see preceding page) built on 432 Hz, the frequency for each pitch on the grid is reduced or enlarged by the number 9. This number is encoded in the mathematics of the universe in that the geometry suggested by the angle sums in this factor 9 grid are webbed into sacred geometry, the geometry of our natural world. Furthermore, we find that these geometric shapes have sound if we convert the sum of angles in the geometric shapes to Hertz (cycles per second) to represent them as pitches.[13]

For example, a basic triangle has 60-degree angles in each of its three corners. Added together, we have 180 degrees, which in terms of frequency is 180 Hz or an F# pitch.

Let us consider a circle with 360 degrees. In pitch, that would be 360 Hz, which is, yes, another F#. The square contains four 90-degree corners, adding up to 360 degrees, or another F#.

Continuing along these same lines, a pentagon has five angles that add up to 540 degrees, or 540 Hz, which is a C#— an overtone of F#. The hexagon is 720 Hz, another F#. A tetrahedron is 720 degrees, again F#. A hexahedron is 2160 degrees, or C#—again one of the overtones of F#. An octahedron is F# again! And lastly, an icosahedron is 3600

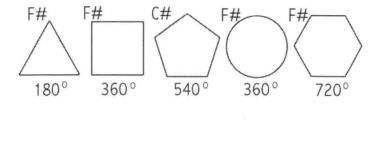

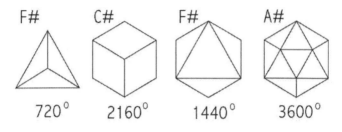

Figure 5.9. Geometric shapes correlating with the musical pitches that form the F# major triad over several octaves.

degrees, or an A#, which, with the C#, completes the F# major triad.

The F# major triad sound reflects *all* the two-dimensional and three-dimensional shapes in the platonic solids. And we can hear them *all* in the F# major triad. Interestingly, by being bathed in the sound of the F# major triad, we are saturating our body in the vibrations of these sacred shapes found throughout nature. I have found that when I play the F# major triad with my crystal bowls, which are tuned to 432 Hz, many people report a "booster rocket" feeling in their consciousness. As a sound healer, I must always take note of the subjective physical and psychological experience of my audience.

An explanation for this expansion of consciousness is that we can see that every geometric shape represented within the flower of life pattern is also perfectly represented by the F# major triad based on the factor 9 grid of 432 Hz. The flower of life is formed by consecutively adding circles one on top of the other. Note that each small circle is a seed of life.

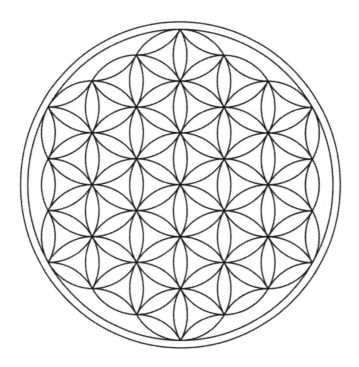

Figure 5.10. Layers of circles forming the flower of life pattern.

In defense of using A432 as a central and basic tone with which to tune musical instruments (as opposed to A440), I would like to offer the fact that if we use 440 Hz as the A in a frequency grid, not one geometry shape would be represented within the grid. Not one. An A at 440 Hz and music tuned to this frequency is entirely inconsistent with natural geometry.

To say that I am in love with the F♯ major triad would be an understatement. In studying the corresponding pitches of the chakras, we find that the heart chakra resonates at F and the throat chakra at G. The high heart (aka the thymus gland) chakra, located between the heart and throat, resonates at F♯. The high heart F♯ chakra connects our consciousness with the sacred geometry of the unified field that surrounds us. I have experienced this miracle of connection countless times.

When I have been extremely stressed, I play the F♯ track from my collaborative composition *Icaros: Chakra Soundscapes* (composed with Daniel Wyman). Depending on my level of stress, this piece has reduced me to tears of relief as I feel my body and spirit re-center. The tears are always from gratitude for the precious gift of the music. I feel connected to myself again. Subjectively, as I listen to the notes of the music I feel my body expressing as more energy and less matter, more wave than particle.

Natural Frequencies of Planets

Although space is a virtual vacuum, we can decipher sound present in the vastness. Yes, sound needs the medium of air or water to travel through, but if we decode electromagnetic vibrations emanating from each of the planets in our solar system we can literally hear the "music of the spheres." The space probe Voyager was sent into space with technology that could record these electromagnetic vibrations as digital information.[14] Sent back to Earth and decoded it can now be heard as intriguing and beautiful sounds from space.

The sounds of the planets are beautiful in an eerie kind of way. After listening to all of them, my favorites are Jupiter (sounding notes C# and E) and Pluto, which hums at a consistent C. The complex interaction of the cosmic plasma of the universe, charged electromagnetic particles from the solar winds and the planetary rings, creates planetary soundscapes that are strangely familiar. Some of their sounds remind me of human voices, whale songs, giant Tibetan singing bowls, and certainly, wind sweeping across a desert. All of this is unexplainable. Once again, the holographic nature of creation is gifted to our ears.

The Schumann Resonances

Our planet has a core resonance and rhythm, which must have played a profound part in the evolution of life. We just don't live on Planet Earth, we live inside her energy, within the unique cavity between the Earth's surface and the ionosphere above us. This frequency, known as the Schumann resonance after the man who detected its presence, is a description of a fundamental resonance of 7.83 Hz, which is caused by sound vibrating within this space.

This space is a resonant cavity within which electromagnetic waves peak and wane.

Truth be told, a spectrum of frequencies may be heard that varies from 3–60 Hz. But 7.83 Hz is the fundamental frequency. Think of this chamber as being a large sphere encircling our planet in which pulses can travel. The Earth is interacting with all living organisms living inside her expansive field. You could refer to the fundamental Schumann resonance as a planetary drummer, or cadence keeper, as we are at its effect all the time. Everything we do is carried out within this soup of entraining energy pulses created by the Earth and her atmosphere and acts like a kind of electrical generator.

Discovered in 1957, Winfried Schumann mathematically calculated this pulse to be around 7.83 Hz. Remembering that our hearing ranges from 20–20,000 Hz, this resonant pitch is far below what we can hear organically; however, we easily can be entrained to this frequency, which lies precisely in the middle frequency where alpha brainwaves and theta brainwave ranges meet. This means that 7.83 is a brainwave frequency of deep relaxation.

It is no wonder that a walk in the forest or a day lying on the beach listening to the waves is healing and restorative. Mother Earth is entraining us to a brainwave frequency of wholeness.

Numerous studies have shown that psychic phenomena and geomagnetic activity have a strong correlation, such that it might be that the Earth's magnetic field serves as a kind of "psychic information highway" or "psychic Internet." The following quote from psi researcher Lian Sidorov is notable:

> For a decade, Robert Beck researched the brainwave activity of healers from all cultures and religious backgrounds (he studied psychics, shamans, dowsers, Christian healers, seers, ESP readers, Hawaiian kahuna, Santeria practitioners, Wicca practitioners, and others). Independent of their belief systems, each exhibited "nearly identical EEG signatures" during their "healing" moments: a 7.8–8 Hz brainwave activity, which lasted from one to several seconds and which was phase and frequency-synchronized with the earth's geoelectric micropulsations, the Schumann resonance.[15]

So, if you want to peer into the future, or perfect your healing techniques, go take a forest "bath."

·····································

SIX

PHYSICAL AND EMOTIONAL IMPACTS
OF HEALING SOUND AND MUSIC

The mainstream medical community is beginning to recognize and utilize alternative therapies such as music and sound therapy. As data-collecting technology is becoming more sensitive to energetic physical changes, the results are being quantified. No longer in the realm of immeasurable results from alternative therapies, we are now entering the age of solid data. My daughter is a medical doctor who uses these therapies in her family practice clinic and her patients benefit greatly from them.

Heart and Brain Coherence

What does *coherence* mean? The term has been used to describe social, physiological, psychological, global, heart, and brain states. *Coherence* refers to orderly, harmonious connectedness and logical states of mind. If a person is coherent, he or she is making sense. When referring to heart and brain coherence, we find that the interrelationship is webbed as well as cyclical, as each organ is always responding to the other.

If you are in a state of coherence, your psycho-physiological state, as measured by indicators in the nervous system, cardiovascular system, hormonal system, and immune system, is running efficiently. All the systems are working together in a coordinated manner to support your health and wellbeing.

How is this optimal state created? Research at the HeartMath Institute has found that the pattern of your heart rhythm displays the emotional state and nervous system markers.[1] This pattern is known as your *heart rate variability* (HRV).

When you are feeling anxious, angry, or tense, your HRV becomes very disordered, or *incoherent.* It is both directly influenced by your emotional state and driven by your thoughts. The brain perceives danger (reflected by emotions of anxiety) and the heart responds, which further causes the brain to begin the cascade or chemical responses of stress. The two feed on each other creating a loop of incoherence.[2]

On the other hand, if the heart and brain are in coherence, the HRV signal appears as an ordered and smooth pattern. In coherence, our physiological systems are in perfect order and there is synchronization. Heart coherence is achieved when positive emotions, such as love and gratitude, are present as opposed to chaos created by fear or anxiety.

In coherence, the brain and the heart function in lockstep, synchronizing in a most intense and deep way. The quickest way to achieve coherence is through the intentional creation of positive feelings. We cannot indulge in the luxury of a negative emotion, as it is like drinking poison. Last week this lesson was driven home to me in a most distinct way. I was driving in heavy traffic during the San Antonio rush hour and minding my own business, being a respectful driver. However, a truck pulled right in front of me, causing me to slam on my brakes and massively disrupting my reveries. Something snapped inside me, and a stream of invective words directed to the driver of the truck flowed out of my mouth. The truck then took off at a high rate of speed, and (again, no thought involved) I followed it, aggressively honking all the way to shame the driver and demonstrate how mad he had made me. We got up to a speed of 80 M.P.H. before I came to my senses and slowed down.

By the end of this episode, my body was flooded with stress hormones and I am sure that my HRV would look like a million spikes of nasty spears if it were displayed on a monitor. Adrenaline must have been coating my every cell with its goo because I was left exhausted. The truck driver could have cared less and went his merry way. I was left thinking, *WHAT JUST HAPPENED?*

This was an exquisite example of incoherence and how quickly it can happen. I know that my response had to do with my perceived reaction of justice against a rude driver, but maybe I was wrong. Maybe the driver had a major emergency and had to get to a hospital. I have no idea. This is an example of how I made an assumption that the driver was rude. Maybe the driver was trying to save a life. Here's the thing: in that moment I could have chosen my response, and I just went with anger without tempering my reaction. For this, I paid the price. It was a lesson for me, someone who should have known better. I think the whole experience would have been different if I had been listening to music, which I was not. I find that music keeps me calm in traffic and cools my brain.

Let us explore that soothing effect.

Some intriguing studies have been done by the researcher at the HeartMath Institute whom we've met in earlier chapters. Dr. Rollin McCraty and his colleagues Mike Atkinson, Glen Rein, and Alan Watkins have investigated the effects of music on heart/brain coherence. Their study "Music Enhances the Effect of Positive Emotional States on Salivary IgA" showed that:

Music can be designed to enhance the beneficial effects of positive emotional states on immunity, and that this effect may be mediated by the autonomic nervous system. This data raises the tantalizing possibility that music and emotional self-management may have significant health benefits in a variety of clinical situations in which there is immunosuppression and autonomic imbalance.[3]

Remember that IgA is immunoglobulin A, an antibody found in the mucous membranes that kills microbes.

Physicist and meditation educator, John Hagelin, Ph.D., who is affiliated with Maharishi University and Transcendental Meditation, has presented research findings on the effects of meditation on the brain and intelligence. His studies find positive effects of meditation on brain coherence and an increase in intelligence. Dr. Hagelin found that after three months of twice-daily meditation the whole brain begins to function coherently, giving rise to increased intelligence, creativity, enhanced learning ability, memory, psychological stability, and emotional maturity, as the frontal lobes become activated.[4]

Hagelin has also found that daily meditation in maximum-security prisons shows a marked reduction in the recidivism rate of inmates.[5] In children with attention deficit hyperactivity disorder (ADHD), meditation shows a profound reversal and elimination of symptoms like the inability to focus and give attention. He showed that the condition is partly caused by the underdevelopment of the prefrontal cortex.[6] The same study showed that the symptoms of ADHD abated as the brain became coherent after twelve weeks of twice daily meditation.[7]

It has been said that the main goal of meditation is to quiet the mind and turn down the "thought machine." Many people find it difficult to achieve that calm state. The easiest way I have found is to listen to music that incorporates binaural beats to create a brainwave state of alpha or theta. Binaural beats are a beat patterns created within the brain through sonic forcing. The beats entrain the brain to specific brainwave patterns. This phenomenon is discussed later in this chapter. The music must be very slow in tempo and fairly constant in volume. The point is to create an aural landscape of peace and consistency.

To allow the heart to entrain to this rhythm and also keep the mind focused on feelings of compassion and gratitude is the quickest and easiest way to enter heart-brain coherence. I feel that it is necessary to do this every day to begin to exist in this coherent state consistently. With practice, this state of calm gratitude and acceptance becomes the normal state, as opposed to normalizing a state of anxiety and stress.

I can attest to the occasional attraction of stress states, as I feel energized and goal oriented by them, BUT leading a constantly stress-laden life is exhausting and physical harmful.

Begin to train your mind by listening to soothing music at least twice a day in a relaxed way to return to a naturally coherent state.

Elimination of Stress Responses

Life can be stressful, whether the stress is work related and short term or has to do with persistent worry about a family situation. Both short-term and long-term stress triggers a cascade of hormones that strongly affect the body and mind. The stress response—or more accurately, a pattern of biochemical responses—has been called the *fight-or-flight response* because it readies the body to escape or defend when it senses a threat. This can be a very positive reaction when we are faced with life-threatening situations, like confronting an oncoming car or imminent danger on the battlefield. The heart begins to pound and the breathing speeds up as our muscles tense in preparation for responding to the threat. In the short term, this response can save our lives.

But if the physiological state continues, as it would in places where the "battle" never ends, a city in a war-torn country with frequent bombings, such as Aleppo, Syria, for example, it can be detrimental to health. The long-term effect of chronic stress causes the release of chemical messengers, like cortisol and adrenaline, which elevate blood pressure and blood sugar and suppress the immune system. Chronic stress has been shown to contribute to anxiety, depression, and addiction. If the glands that produce the hormones are triggered too often, they become unable to function, which is why adrenal fatigue is part of this picture of constant stress. We can also run out of sufficient neurotransmitters for normal brain functions. It takes time to regenerate our resources after confronting stress. Rest and nourishment are key.

We have two nervous systems that direct chemical and neurochemical release to manage our physiological states. These systems are under the control of the autonomic nervous system, which acts unconsciously to regulate physiological functions like heart rate, digestion, respiratory rate, and eye pupil dilation. This system, which is also in control of the fight-or-flight response, is managed by two different players or directors: the *sympathetic nervous system* (which activates it) and the *parasympathetic nervous system* (which deactivates it).

When stimulated by thought, the sympathetic nervous system can accelerate heart rate, widen bronchial passages, decrease motion within the large intestine, constrict blood vessels, and raise blood pressure. This cascade of physiological reactions is caused when the two amygdalae in the brain (one in each hemisphere) are warned of danger and send signals to the hypothalamus. The hypothalamus contacts the adrenal glands in the torso, and there is a release of adrenaline, which is like the gas pedal to the body to gear up either for a flight or a fight.

Heart rate increases, blood pressure goes up, and the person begins to breathe more rapidly as small airways in the lungs open up.

Once the danger is past, the parasympathetic system takes over and acts like a brake. It signals the body to return to homeostasis and calm. It signals the body to *rest and digest.*

An example that I find most appropriate is that of a grazing zebra on the Serengeti Plain in Tanzania. If the zebra sees a lion closing in for a kill, its stress response is kicked into full gear and the zebra runs for his life to escape the predator. This escape requires intense muscular support from the zebra's body.

Luckily, the zebra escapes the lion. Now he immediately returns to grazing with the rest of his fortunate friends, and, as the danger passes, his parasympathetic system returns him and the scene to one of peace and calm. Once again, the sun sets tranquilly on the Serengeti.

However, if a person (not a zebra) has constant thoughts of danger or anxiety, the stress response become chronic. Disease is not far away as a result of the elevated stress state. All is NOT peaceful or tranquil in that landscape.

Unfortunately, many people become habituated to the feeling of stress and don't recognize the dangers of cortisol and adrenaline saturating their bodies in a constant flow. Because the body has a hard time telling the difference between real danger and perceived danger the response is always the same.

An acronym that is helpful when learning to reduce mental stress is FEAR or *false evidence appearing real.* We must not always believe what the mind tells us is scary.

I have an experiment for you right now to prove how powerful an inventor your mind is and how your body believes what you think. Imagine a lemon in your hand. Actually, hold your hand out in front of you with the imaginary lemon on it. The lemon is cut in half and you have one half in your hand. It is cold, and the juice is dripping down the side of the yellow peel of the lemon. Now bring your hand up to your mouth with the lemon on it and take a bite of the lemon.

What happened to your salivary glands? I would guess that you started to salivate with just the imagination of a lemon. Actually, even as I wrote this, I started to salivate. Crazy, huh? *That* is how powerful our thoughts are.

So, be very aware of how you think, as your body will believe everything you think and respond accordingly to it. When you are at work, there is no lion waiting to take you down. You may think that there is one, or an equivalent, but remember that thoughts can be false and untrue.

One very easy way to return your thoughts and body to calm is to listen to music that is slow and meditative. As your mind slows down, your body will follow, and you will be in a state of healing and creative flow. Listen to music at work . . . be like the grazing zebra. Rest and digest.

Brainwave States and Healing

Brainwaves are wavelike patterns generated by the individual cells of the brain (*neurons*), which communicate with each other through electrical changes and charges. We see these electrical changes in an electroencephalogram (EEG) readout, displayed in the form of brainwaves. The combination of millions of neurons sending electrical signals produces these brainwave pattern, which most often will fall into one of four main brainwave states: delta, theta, alpha, and beta. A fifth state exists: gamma.

In the mid-1920s, German neurologist Hans Berger discovered the existence of brainwaves. Interestingly, Berger's path to this discovery began because he wanted to record what he thought was psychic energy in the brain. Ultimately, he narrowed his study and captured the first recording of electrical waves in the brain with his invention, the EEG, gathering evidence of alpha brainwaves.

We have previously touched upon brainwave states when discussing forced brainwave states or entrainment. Before a deeper exploration of each brainwave state in a healing context, let us ponder the impact of our brainwave signature or profile to our daily experience. Exhaustive research has linked specific brainwave patterns with all manner of emotional and neurological and physical conditions. A predominance of beta brainwaves, for example, has been linked by research with anxiety disorders, sleep problems, hypervigilance, impulsive behavior, and anger/aggression.[8] In general, we are used to being in the beta brainwave state when we are consciously alert. This is not the state of calm, measured thinking. We are very reactive in beta. We are in beta when we feel agitated, stressed, hurried, and pressured. Most drivers on the highway are in beta during rush hour (myself included, as you know). Sadly, it is the dominant brainwave for most of us, most of the time. It wears us out if we cannot shift our brainwaves to something more restful.

When we alter our brainwave rhythm to alpha, we are slowing our brainwaves. The benefit of this is that it puts us in a highly productive brain state. In alpha, we are capable of analyzing complex situations, learning new information quickly, and performing creative tasks with flow. We are less reactive than in beta. Studies have shown that the alpha brainwave state allows for the release of beneficial brain chemicals, such as norepinephrine, endorphins, and dopamine. These neurotransmitters are linked to mental clarity and learning.

Let me now describe the five brainwave states in detail, beginning with the slowest, deepest state, and then I'll explain how a sound healer would make use of them.

DELTA WAVES (0.5 TO 3 Hertz)
Deep Sleep

Delta is the slowest band of waves that our brains produce, and they occur when we are in deep, dreamless sleep. These waves are very beneficial for the body, which restores and heals itself in this state. The delta state releases antiaging hormones, including melatonin and DHEA. Human growth hormone (HGH) is another antiaging hormone that is increased when delta brainwaves are occurring inside the brain, due to the stimulation of the pituitary gland. HGH maintains the skin, bone density, cartilage, and the joints in the body, as well as speeds up the healing process of joint and cartilage injuries. Delta is the brainwave state of deepest relaxation, deepest healing, deepest spiritual connection, and deepest connection with the subconscious mind. This state is considered to be the gateway to the unconscious mind and the collective unconscious.

THETA WAVES (3 TO 8 HZ)
Deep Relaxation and Trance

Theta brainwaves occur most often in deep meditation. In theta, our physical senses are withdrawn from the external world and our awareness is focused on signals from within our psyche.

Theta brainwave states have been the goal for those who meditate for centuries. It is common for people to feel as if they are in a trance, where the mind feels as though it may have gone to sleep, although it is vaguely aware of what is happening around it. Theta gives us a capacity for prolonged daydreaming, where a loss of time may be experienced. My clients who experience sound therapy listen to music that induces the theta state. They routinely say, "I went away. I left my body. I was asleep, but not really. I saw things I never knew existed." All such statements are reports of experiences while in the theta state. In theta, we also enjoy whole-brain functioning, as in the alpha state. We are synchronized in mind, body, and spirit.

ALPHA WAVES (8 TO 12 HZ)
Relaxation and Daydreams

Alpha brainwaves are dominant during quietly flowing thoughts, and in some meditative states. Alpha is the "power of now," of being alert in the present. Alpha is the restorative resting state, which is highly creative for the brain.

Alpha brainwaves signal states of daydreaming and fantasizing, relaxation, and detached awareness. For example, close your eyes and imagine a sunset against the ocean. See the sun setting below the horizon and hear the seagulls flying low near the shore. You have begun to induce an alpha state. This technique has been used in guided meditations and shamanic journeys. Alpha also has been known to lower the experience of physical pain and therefore is useful in healing as stress is reduced.

The benefits of this state are numerous. Our brain hemispheres become synchronized as in the theta state. There is reduced anxiety, reduction of chronic pain, high blood pressure, and increase in energy and happiness.

Other ways to induce the alpha state are doing light housework, taking a shower, or engaging in routine tasks, like gardening. Painting pictures can induce the alpha state. I have a friend who suggested that her husband take up painting as a way to balance his busy and stressful life as a doctor. He loved the time he spent with a paintbrush so much that he continued this hobby well into his eighties. I am sure that the relaxed alpha state he enjoyed extended his life, as he had an autoimmune disease. Interestingly, whenever he painted, he was disease free. His mind traveled to the beautiful places that were emerging from his canvas and he lived as a healthy strong man in those exotic landscapes.

BETA WAVES (12 TO 38 HZ)
Normal Waking Consciousness

Whenever you are thinking, talking, and communicating, your mind is producing beta waves. Beta is the state in which you are active and alert; and it is the most common brainwave pattern we experience. Generally, the left hemisphere of the brain is engaged when we are engaged in mental activity. When beta wave activity is very intense, our hemispheres become much less synchronized, as this is the wave state needed for the fight-or-flight response. A chronic beta state leads to anxiety, stress, worry, fear, and insomnia. With this state, a cascade of neurochemicals is released by the adrenal glands, triggering the fight-or-flight, stress response.

When we need heightened awareness, it is available to us. But if this heightened awareness is a constant state, we are at risk for disease, both physical and mental. Adrenal fatigue is a common complaint of people in high-stress jobs. A mild form of adrenal insufficiency caused by chronic stress leads to this condition. It is thought that the adrenal glands are unable to continue to function in a healthy way as the constant fight-or-flight arousal and beta state taxes the adrenals beyond the limits of healthy functioning. As a result, their function becomes limited and fatigue is a result.

GAMMA WAVES (38 TO 42 HZ with capacity to reach 5,000 cycles a second) Higher Mental Activity

Gamma brainwaves are the most rapid in frequency of any brainwaves. They signal our induction into a brainwave state that is able to process large amounts of information and link information from all parts of the brain in a small amount of time.

Interestingly, the gamma wave is above the frequency of neuronal firing—so how these cycles per second are generated is not yet clearly understood. Tibetan Buddhist monks reach this state consistently and report expanded consciousness and spiritual emergence.

Experiments on meditating Tibetan Buddhist monks using brain-scanning technology have shown a correlation between transcendental mental states and gamma waves. The 2004 study "Long-term Meditators Self-induce High-amplitude Gamma Synchrony during Mental Practice" conducted at the Brain Imaging Lab and the Center for Investigating Healthy Minds at the Waisman Center at the University of Wisconsin, Madison, by Antoine Lutz, Ph.D., the late Lawrence L. Greischar, Ph.D., Nancy B. Rawlings, D.Phil., Matthieu Ricard, Ph.D. (a Buddhist monk who has been called the World's Happiest Man), and Richard Davidson, Ph.D., took eight longtime practitioners of Buddhist meditation, and, using electrodes, monitored the patterns of electrical activity produced by their brains as they meditated.[9]

For a control, the researchers compared the brain activity of the monks to a group of novice meditators. In a normal meditative state, both groups were shown to have similar brain activity. However, when the monks were told to generate an objective feeling of compassion during meditation, their brain activity displayed a frequency of 40 Hz, the rhythm of gamma waves.[10] By focusing on compassion and love, it is possible to train the brain to produce more gamma brainwave activity, hence induce whole-brain coherence.

How to Alter Brainwaves Using Sound: Binaural Beats and Isochronic Beats

You can train your brain to change its waves by learning meditation and relaxation techniques. However, it can take weeks, and, for some people, even years, to experience the powerful benefits of brainwave entrainment through meditation alone. Fortunately, there is a shortcut to getting the best from your brainwaves—using audio tones to produce what are known as *binaural beats*. Binaural beats can effectively entrain and synchronize your brainwaves to any brainwave pattern you want to experience.

Binaural beats work by sending a different frequency to each ear. When hearing the two frequencies at the same time, the brain creates a third tone at the frequency that is the mathematical difference between the two. For example, if a 310 Hz frequency is sent to the left ear and a 315 Hz frequency is sent to the right ear, the brain will process and create a third frequency—in this case, 5 Hz. The brain then entrains to this frequency of 5 Hz and produces brainwave patterns that align with it. In this case, the brain would slip into a theta wave pattern effortlessly.

It usually takes about five minutes of hearing the two pitches for the brain to fully respond. The technical term for this is *frequency following response.*

On the other hand, many people enjoy music which uses *isochronic beats* to create a desired brainwave state. In this case, only one sound is used, repeatedly pulsing at the rate of five cycles per second. In Greek, *iso* means "one" and *chronic* means "constantly recurring." In other words, the beat is repeating over and over. We saw this earlier when we discussed how shamanic drumming creates forced brainwave states.

I find from my own experience that isochronic beats are not as effective for brainwave entrainment in the lower frequency ranges of delta and theta.[11] I use binaural beat meditation music exclusively, as the repeated note in isochronic beats can be distracting, which is not an emotion I want created in me while I meditate. However, I know that shamanic practitioners will use isochronic beats for experiences called *journeys*, in which they travel to other dimensions of reality to commune with ancestral spirits and spirit guides. Some anecdotally report that the beating creates a sense of urgency that is helpful in making the passage through the barriers to these subtle dimensions.

Binaural beat music is extremely effective and can increase your creative energy, improve sleep, or generally help with focus. There is a veritable wonderland of music available to choose from that uses binaural beats to assist in focus, studying or deep meditation. Find something you like and see how it affects your own productivity.

Connection to Soul, Spirit, and Source with Sound

As sound makers, sound lovers, music experiencers, and music magicians, we have a sacred duty to express our highest potential as souls. The following are reflections I have that address this journey in myriads of ways. Not all the paths I traveled were full of love and light, but all were rich in life lessons.

In the early part of my life, I spent a great deal of time searching for happiness, love, and peace. I looked to others and the outer world for the source of these elusive and precious gifts. The truth is that love, peace, truth, and happiness cannot be found. They cannot be gained or earned. They cannot be taught. They cannot be learned from books or priests, organizations, and workshops. They are all released from our own hearts, minds, and consciousness, where they have resided from inception. These beautiful qualities ARE us, so we cannot find them, but must become and uncover them. Music offered me a bridge to begin to view and acquaint myself with these beautiful qualities. It offered me a path in.

I matured into knowing that consciousness must change and transcend until all that is unloving and untruthful and fearful falls away. Then, and only then, would I be capable of expressing peace, truth, love, and happiness. Then I could fully embody those qualities, which I was seeking. Love is never found, it is embodied by each soul.

Truth is never found.

Happiness is never found.

Embodiment of the positive qualities of experience so fervently sought is a "becoming," a "transformation," and an "awakening." It arises in the consciousness as the soul evolves. And, just as the beautiful butterfly emerges from her cocoon, free to fly, with her wings spread to the sun, so each soul becomes free to be the happiness and joy he or she so desperately searched for. Now, the spiritual pilgrim just "is" this happiness, this love, this peace.

Once this happens, there is no need for rules, dogma, direction, or control because the soul can only act from its deepest reality: the state of love and unity. A peach can only express "peachness" because that is what it is, a peach. It is not a thorn. It cannot be anything other than itself. Quiet and deep, the evolved pilgrim, like the peach, expresses himself or herself as a living embodiment of that deepest reality of love and compassion. The search is over. What was so desperately yearned for was always there. The aspirant has emerged and has become free. I was free.

I finally understood that I could use music to bring compassion to my heart and healing waves to my brain. I began to see everything through the eyes of love and my dream became beautiful. As I began to dwell within the love consciousness of music I began to hear the constantly singing chorus of love that was playing in the background of my life. Once I perceived it, my entire life became a dance of gratitude and a song of joy. Every movement was a dance and every word became a song. Certainly, there were times when I forgot and lost touch with the music, but the feelings of loneliness and separation drove me back to gratitude and I was once again in the connected flow.

Music can be used to evoke this gratitude, love, and compassion—healing states of being. By making use of sound and music to heal ourselves, we become masters of our own reality.

Up-Regulation of Genetic and Cellular Influences Using Music

Joe Dispenza, D.C., author of *Becoming Supernatural: How Common People Are Doing the Uncommon,* has made a profound impact on the meditation and medical communities over the last ten years. His research has shown the profound influence of thoughts on genetic expression. He states:

All genes do is make proteins, which are responsible for the structure and function of your body. Your immune system makes immune proteins called antibodies, your skin cells make skin proteins called collagen, and your stomach cells make proteins called enzymes. For a cell to make a protein, a gene has to be regulated. We have 100,000 proteins that make up our body plus about 40,000 that regulate and assist the body to make those 100,000 proteins—so we have 140,000 proteins total. That means we should have 140,000 genes, but it turns out that we only have 23,688. So, we have more proteins than genes. The epigenetics model states that we can have different variations on the same gene—as many as 35,000, in fact.

Genes up-regulate or turn on and produce healthy proteins, or they down-regulate or shut off and produce modified or unhealthy proteins. As long as you keep thinking, acting, and feeling the same way, you keep the same genes turned on and the other genes turned off—and now you're headed for your genetic destiny.

As you begin to modify your thoughts, behaviors, and emotional states, you can turn on thousands of different gene expressions that begin to make new proteins. Certain genes are more actively signaled than others but again, the stronger the signal, the more profound the experience; the more altered the behavior, the more we change our genetic expression. Our nervous system is actually the greatest pharmacy in the world[12]

Dr. Dispenza teaches his readers many methods to shift their thinking and allow the emergence of a new personality, free from the limiting beliefs of the past. One of the most powerful ways I myself have found to modify thoughts and emotional states is making and listening to music. The body frequency, through music, is raised to the frequency of love and compassion, which is a very fast, rarified frequency.

For healing to occur, the connection to the unified field must be solid and consistent, as an opening of the heart follows, and thus, heart and brain coherence is generated. Energy must flow out of the heart chakra (fourth energy center), as a state of oneness and wholeness. Remember, the heart chakra resonates with the pitch of F. At the heart level, there is a deep connection to the quantum or unified field, facilitating the achievement of the state we call zero-point awareness—awareness of the infinite potential of the quantum field. As this happens, polarity and duality move into oneness.

When the heart center is fully activated, personal awareness moves within and the individual become more energy than matter, more light than physical structure, more wave than particle. Then one has entered the field of all possibility without limitation.

When the heart opens, connection to the soul is felt. It is like coming home to peace after a long, awkward journey through a terrifying land. This is the home state in which the body can heal by up-regulating the healing genes and down-regulating the destructive genes.

Neurochemical Balance Achieved Through Meditative Music

Meditation and mindfulness both signify a mental state that is reached by focusing attention on the present moment. Many people enjoy this practice by focusing on breathing while calmly observing their thoughts and accepting their transient flow. Bringing their awareness back to the act of breathing slowly brings their attention to the present moment. Slowly the realization unfolds in their consciousness that mental "chatter" simply comes and goes, and the only true reality is the present moment.

We find that meditation or contemplative prayer is supported by all the major world religions—Hinduism, Buddhism, Judaism, Islam, and Christianity. Saying the rosary or repeating a mantra are two examples of current tools used to reach a meditative state. Meditators can achieve mental states of deep peace and acceptance with training, and, sometimes, years of practice.

Personally, I have always found this kind of meditation to be almost beyond my ability to achieve. My active mind takes over my brain and it jumps from topic to topic. Through binaural beat music, I have found a way to reach these deep states of awareness easily and with great success. Reaching these states has proven to be extremely beneficial for my health. As I explained in an earlier chapter, I found that my anxiety lessened. Also, my sleep improved. As an effect of binaural beat music, others have report experiencing relief from depression, a decrease is reactive behavior, and being better able to manage addictive urges.

The key to all such improvements is the release and management of neurochemicals within the brain. Meditation has been shown by countless studies to increase serotonin, DHEA, GABA, endorphins, and melatonin, and to control cortisol, which is a result of stress.

Let us look at the benefits by exploring the different neurochemicals released by the brain during these deep states of meditation.

Serotonin

Serotonin has a profound impact on our moods and feelings of wellbeing. It is known as the "happy" neurotransmitter. In the *Journal of Psychiatry and Neuroscience,* Simon N. Young reports that meditation is a practice that can influence the release of this neurochemical.[13] It seems that the release of serotonin is directly linked to feelings of peace. In effect, the two are in a loop. More feelings of peace create more serotonin and more serotonin creates feelings of peace.

DHEA

The modern-day fountain of youth is DHEA, or the "youth hormone." It is known as the longevity molecule in antiaging circles. As we age, DHEA levels in our bodies decrease and aging ensues with all its attendant diseases. DHEA is a hormone that is a precursor to the sex hormones testosterone and estrogen. As those hormones decline, degenerative aging and disease can follow. Vincent Giampapa, M.D., former president and founding member of the American Board of Anti-Aging Medicine, has discovered that meditation practitioners have 43.77 percent more DHEA than nonmeditators in the same age group.[14] DHEA benefits energy, muscle tone, fat loss, and inflammation in the body, to name a few body functions.

GABA

People with addiction challenges can benefit greatly by meditation. Apparently, GABA (gamma aminobutyric acid) is the "calm" neurotransmitter. Anyone with an addiction to alcohol, drugs, tobacco, or food is likely to have a distinct deficit of GABA. Not having enough of this chemical can create anxiety, nervousness, and poor sleep. In 2010, psychiatrists at the Boston University School of Medicine found a 27 percent increase in GABA after sixty minutes of yoga.[15] True, yoga is not traditional meditation but could be considered moving meditation. That is a remarkable finding and could prove to be of great benefit to those suffering with addictions.

Endorphins

We are all familiar with the phrase "runner's high," which describes the euphoria that runners have after a long run. The neurotransmitter release of endorphins causes this well reported state of wellbeing. In 1995, a study published in *Biological Psychology Journal* tested the endorphin release in two groups of people, runners and meditators. Surprisingly, in both groups the endorphin levels were elevated.[16]

Endorphins have a positive effect on motivation, relaxation, stress relief, and wellbeing. We all know people who seem "addicted" to physical fitness activities, such as running or bicycling. They crave the endorphin release, and these activities prove to be very beneficial for them. Physical stress and the predictable release of adrenaline comes with vigorous exercise, A release of endorphins is the subsequent relief they gain from self-medicating with running. I guess it works. No judgment here, as I have my favorite "medicines" too, which is performing or drinking a glass of wine after a hard day of work.

Melatonin

Jet lag? Melatonin to the rescue. Certainly, many have used this critical chemical to get much-needed rest after a trip across the United States through four time zones. On one of my trips to sing in China, I was ever so grateful for the melatonin tablets I took to help regulate my sleep patterns and sync with Chinese time zones.

Also, with the fairly new invention of electric lights we have altered our production of melatonin, which is linked to cessation of light. Our light-filled days have become longer and our nights shorter, contributing to our dysregulation of sleep. *Fun fact:* In 1925, only half the homes in America had electric power.

Melatonin is produced by the pineal gland, which releases this neurochemical as the light in the environment decreases (nighttime). That is why it is important to sleep in a dark room—light tends to stop the production of this very important chemical. We pay with a large biological toll if we are not exposed to darkness, as melatonin protects us from cancer and strengthens the immune system. Meditation can boost melatonin levels and can serve as a much-needed balance in our busy lives.

Cortisol

A major stress hormone, cortisol is also a major aging chemical. When we move into the stress response, we produce cortisol and adrenaline, and, for a short time, this benefits us. However, if we are constantly bathed in these chemicals, our bodies begin to break down, which leads to anxiety, inflammation, and depression. To make matters worse, cortisol also blocks the creation of beneficial hormones.

Recent research from the Shamatha Project at the University of California, Davis, conducted by Clifford Saron, Ph.D., and a team of doctoral and postdoctoral researchers, has just come forward. They found that focusing on the present through meditation lowered the levels of the stress hormone, cortisol.[17] "This is the first study to show a direct relation between resting cortisol and scores on any type of mindfulness scale"[18] said Tonya Jacobs, a postdoctoral researcher and first author of a paper describing the study. We do have a powerful tool to combat the effects of stress and cortisol levels.

SEVEN

IMPLEMENTING SOUND AS A HEALING AGENT

I have been in love with sound since I emerged into this world. My mother said that she could remember the little songs I would sing to myself as a toddler. I would make up songs about baby birds, kitties, flowers, and all manner of child-world critters. My mother also said that rather than cry as a child, I would howl in pitches, and thus began my early career as an opera singer. This career was certainly a dream unfulfilled for many years, but from the beginning of my life I was experimenting with sounding my emotions and my reactions to the world.

Toning

Sound, I have come to understand, is a way to express and process feelings, emotions, and reactions to events that we cannot put into words. We laugh when we are so overcome with joy that the exuberance explodes into gales of sound. We cry, sometimes very loudly and uncontrollably, when the grief is beyond our ability to hold it in our bodies. We shout when we become angry or are moved to depths of indignation or frustration. We sing when we are grieving, worshipping, comforting, consoling, rejoicing, and working. We sing by ourselves and in groups. Each kind of singing offers a different and rich experience for the singer/sounder.

As a vocal soloist, I sang with symphonies, choruses, popular music band, and folk singer (with my guitar). As a mom, I sang with my young daughter. As a grade school teacher, I sang with my music classes. As a university vocal professor, I sang with my students. Today, I sing with my sound therapy clients and I sing my own compositions for voice and piano. I sing when I do sound baths for audiences who have come for healing and immersion in sonic waves that can realign their chakras. My entire life has been filled with vocal sound. I took it for granted that the balance in my body and soul was normal and that this balance was available to everyone. After all, everybody can sing, can't they?

But I learned a very valuable lesson in what "no singing" felt like after I severely shattered my shoulder into pieces while falling from my horse. For six weeks, I did not sing, cry, or utter much sound at all. Most of the time, I was on such dulling pain medication that I don't remember much. I do, however, remember feeling only half awake in my body, as if it was struggling to just keep me functioning. I remember feeling deadness at my core. Who knows what that was, but I do know that when I began to sing again, the deadness disappeared. I felt alive again and revitalized from the inside out. What I missed and what I needed to do was to produce vocal sound and frequency in my body daily. I had gotten used to feeling alive inside by the vocal sounding and singing I experienced throughout my life.

Many books have influenced my knowledge of sounding, but there is one that came at just the right time. Over twenty years ago, I read *Healing Yourself with Your Own Voice* by Don Campbell. In this book, he describes *toning*, a type of vocal sounding on different pitches using just vowels as the breath is released. He claims that he cured a tumor in his head by toning daily. This caught my attention and I experimented with it for a period of time. Being a singer, I originally thought that I already "toned" daily by constantly singing. Not really so, as I ultimately discovered.

Now, as life has a way of morphing into new forms, a new career opened up to me as a sound therapist and heightened my awareness. In reflecting on the benefits of toning and the healing it offers my clients, my memories of Don Campbell's experience resurfaced, and I realized there is a difference between singing and toning. For me, my experiences with the curative benefits of sounding are numerous. By this, I mean that the vibration in my body created by making a vocal sound has brought me either emotional resolution or healing at the physical level.

When my father died, I could not hold the grief in my body. The sound that came out of that grief was of a wounded animal. How could I have held that in? How could I have suppressed that grief? Another example of emotional release through sound came in a workshop for addressing that specific purpose. I released a sound of despair that was profound and so unknown to me but was somehow trapped in the cells of my body. I still don't know what would cause that sound to come forth, but after the sound was released, the physical pain in my back was gone.

Physical pain and discomfort are quickly addressed with our own sounding. When I was in Peru this past year, I had one of the most severe migraine attacks I can remember. I had no medication on hand and it was 2:00 A.M. I was alone in a hotel room and in severe pain. I decided to heal myself (like the old adage "Physician, heal thyself"), so I began to tone. I toned for eight minutes on each pitch of the diatonic C major scale. There are seven pitches, so I settled down for a fifty-six-minute experiment using the syllable AUM.

I began by breathing very deeply into my belly and sounded the AH vowel sound, and slowly moved to OO, and then into a gentle MMM. As I toned, I realized that at least I was not thinking about my pain, because my mind was being given something else to do. Good to know. But about thirty minutes into my toning, I realized that the relief I was experiencing was not just my imagination. The crushing pain was backing off. Hallelujah!

After I finished toning AH-OOH-UMM for all the seven pitches, I was filled with gratitude and peace and went blissfully to sleep. The next morning, I was still migraine free. This was an amazing event for me. This really works!

I have become devoted to daily toning. It is important to note how singing is different from toning. Toning is the sounding of one pitch for an extended period. Singing is many pitches strung together in a lyrical musical line (a melody), which can move much faster than toning. Each type of expression is valuable, but I have discovered the world of toning, apart from singing.

As I continued with this practice over the months that ensued, I realized that the sound produced in my body was creating amazing healing benefits. I felt much calmer as I adjusted to a new normal of the more relaxed brainwave state of alpha that allows for clearer thinking,

I encourage you to begin a daily practice of toning, which is a very easy and effortless sound meditation. It does not matter whether or not you have skill or talent as a singer. If you can talk, you can tone. Toning isn't singing. It is sound making with the intention to create an even and balanced energy flow in the body and a calm state of mind.

The balanced energy comes from stimulating each of the main chakras in the body using specific vowel sounds (specific pitches can be toned, also, but are not necessary), the intake of breath (life energy), and a calm state of mind.

The latter results from holding the intention of peace toward yourself during the toning.

Allow me to walk you through a Toning for Beginners crash course.

Toning for Beginners

In this minicourse, we will address two very large components and then see the smaller expressions within those broad bases. The components are simply: energy and space.

The energetic aspect is breath, intention, and focus.

The space aspect is posture and the resonating cavities created by mouth, throat, chest, and abdomen.

Exercise 1: Belly Breathing

Begin by sitting in a chair with your torso scooted forward to the edge of the seat and your spine held erect. Balance on your tailbones. I want your entire abdomen to be free to expand so you can take a very deep and full breath.

In this posture, place your hands on your belly and take a breath, noticing as your belly expands outward. When some toners begin, they take a high breath, which raises the shoulders and creates tension in the throat area. That should be avoided if you want to get the deepest, most resonant toning sound. (It is also easier to breathe into the belly.) Do these belly breaths five or six times to get the hang of it.

- Take the breath in for a count of five.
- Hold for five counts.
- Then release for a count of eight.
- Rest for six counts.
- And begin again.

You will notice that after a couple of breaths you are beginning to feel calm and relaxed. Your parasympathetic nervous system is coming on line and you are well on your way to be a toning master!

It might help to get the feeling of the deep breath if you totally relax your abdomen and belly before taking in air. The result of relaxing the belly is that this allows the diaphragm to descend and gives you much more space in your lower lungs to take in nourishing air.

As you breathe, you will also feel your lower back expand. Since we know that tension and lower back pain come hand in hand, this expansion is another goodie you will get from toning—a relaxed and pain-free lower back.

OK. You're doing great, I have no doubt. Let's move on to the next physical skill (I will address the more esoteric elements later).

Exercise 2: Toning Vowel Sounds

I want you to feel the space in your mouth. Really open your mouth as if you are going to yawn a very deep yawn. You will notice that your jaw will drop, your soft palate (the soft roof of your mouth in back of the hard roof) will rise, and the throat will open. Go ahead, just yawn now. I just made myself yawn simply writing about it!

You have now opened a very big resonating space that is ready to accept sound.

First, try an AH vowel sound (as in the word *saw*). Take breath into your belly and just say AHHHH in the same mouth space that we just experimented with before the full yawning shape. It doesn't matter what pitch you are sounding. In fact, let the sound slide around to different pitches. I just want you to become acquainted with sound that is not designated as a "word spoken."

Let that AH ride on the breath for about five counts. Right now, you are just sounding. You will receive benefit from this if you just AHHH for a full couple of minutes using the correct breathing. Remember the breath must be deep and full before your AHHH begins to ride on the released breath.

Great. Now you can move on to different vowels. Toning uses different vowels to access the energetic signature of each chakra. This is an experiment to see what happens.

Try sounding an EH sound (as in the word *say*.) Again, I remind you to take the full five count breath in to your belly, and then on the out breath, you will sound the vowel, EH.

Do this multiple times, until it is comfortable.

The next vowel sound to tone is EEE (as in the word *see*). Let the vowel be very, very bright. The outer edges of your tongue will be nearly touching the edges of your back teeth as this vowel is sounded.

Take the breath in on a count of five and let it release with the vowel EE riding on the out-breath. Pay attention to the steady flow of your breath and the sound of the vowel to make sure you keep the breath going and that the vowel stays a pure EE.

Do this repeatedly for about a minute.

Now, you are going to combine the three vowels in a sequence: AH–EH–EE. Begin by breathing in. Then release the air in your lungs, sounding the vowels with a very smooth transition between each of them.

Try this over and over. As you do, you may begin to notice that each vowel is resonating a different part of your body. For me, the AH vowel resonates my solar plexus chakra and heart chakra. The EH moves up to the heart chakra and throat chakra. The EE resonates in the brow chakra and crown chakra.

To reiterate, it is not necessary to tone on a specific pitch to receive great benefits. I have always had complete faith in the wisdom of the body to pick the correct pitch to begin. You may, however, want to experiment with picking a higher or lower pitch after a while just to see if the resonating sensations change in your body. Feel free to explore.

Let's not forget the subtle addition of intention and focus as you tone. Your thoughts carry power . . . great power, so use this power in a directed way to heal yourself. I always ask the spirit of compassion and love to sound through me with a healing and restoring energy as I tone. I bathe myself in divine light riding on the sound I am creating in my body.

Please don't get overwhelmed here. There is no right and wrong way to do this. You are just giving your body an opportunity to express itself through sound. Let it lead you in your toning, as there is much wisdom in the body.

You may find that a certain spot that the toning brings emotions to the surface. I encourage you to follow the thread of those emotions and release them if you can. You will clear and clean your energetic body this way.

Some schools of thought dictate and describe much more complicated approaches to toning, but I have just done what I felt my body wanted to do. "Simple" has worked just fine for me. By overthinking the process, it could become about making it "right," so I want you to approach your toning with an attitude of play and discovery.

You may want to tone a mantra at some point. OM MANI PADME HUM is a profound Tibetan Buddhist mantra that expresses the principal of compassion for all beings. You can spend some time on the MMM to really feel the vibration in your face. Also, the MMM in OM will get you started with definite physical feedback.

It's fun! Enjoy the lovely instrument inside you. We are built to sound and tone. If you really want to get fancy, purchase a crystal singing bowl and tone along with your bowl. Go to a store and try out different pitches of bowls to find one that suits your voice and temperament.

I hope this has helped take the mystery out of toning. It is as natural as sighing, laughing, crying, and humming. If you experience toning as a daily practice, I promise you that you will gain great benefits from the breathwork inherent in toning and the sound as an inner sonic message. Sound and toning can be a great healer, agent for discovery, a sonic bridge into soul, and a compassionate gift to your spirit, mind, and body.

You will love it!

Therapeutic Vocal Sounding and Singing

The body is an energetic system, a matrix of vibrational frequencies. Ideally, it acts in concert with all of its systems with no incongruent actions or conflict. In other words, the body, mind, and spirit vibrate in harmony.

All thought has a vibration. The more positive thoughts vibrate at a higher frequency than the negative thoughts. Joy and love have a very high frequency; and hate, resentment, fear, and bitterness lower frequencies. These thoughts, when generated by an individual become integrated in the body matrix of field frequencies and either encourage flow and dynamic motion or manifest as disease, tension, and constriction.

Trauma and depression introduce a dampening action and cause energy to get stuck, clouded, and become resistant to flow. Thoughts have specific frequency that our cells respond to, which can encourage dynamic flow or destructive constriction. Negative thoughts can cause two things: energetic resistance and constriction (no flow) and/or physical tension. Both of these can be heard in the sound of the spoken voice. A full resonant voice cannot be produced if energetic resistance and/or physical tensions are present.

By using deep full breath and voice sounding (no speech), we can discover how to release natural, unfettered sound that is fully balanced and fully authentic.

Psychological trauma sometimes causes events to be stored in the body and senses. For this to occur, the memory of an event is so traumatic that it bypasses the speech center and is processed by the limbic system and stored as feelings and sensations. At the time of the traumatic event, the brain (especially the neocortex) is flooded with chemicals and the event is downshifted to the limbic system, which is in charge of emotions and the memory of causative events. Thus, cognitive processes are not present in the time of trauma. The person is purely drenched in survival modalities and fighting for survival. Consequently, the event lies in fragments, submerged in the psyche and stored in the body/mind, unreachable by spoken language.

Very often the fragmented trauma is evident in body posture, manner of breathing, quality of spoken voice, eye contact, and rhythm of speech. The subtle release of energy is also an indicator of the level of physiological and physical health. Energy can be withheld, released in spurts, dampened, and also drained on other people. Highly charged, negative energy typically is exploded or drained as a way of release. Clearly, this is not ideal, but that is an example of fragmented negative energy stored in the unconscious which has not been confronted, processed, and integrated.

To contact the fragmented event, we must speak to it in the language with which it was stored: sound, feelings, and physical sensations. By remembering the event using deep breath and sound, we can then slowly move it to the frontal cortex of the brain to be assessed, reordered, and finally integrated by our cognitive processes.

In some cases, it is not even necessary to remember an event, but it must be given a voice to express. Wailing, crying, moaning, screaming is giving voice to the event. If these reactions to the traumatic event were suppressed at the time of the event, the entire body and vocal production suffers from the restriction and compromises the release of energy and sound. Unless the unconscious trauma is confronted, it will continue to cry for attention by acting out in sabotaging behavior, phobias, and personality disorders.

A person is not fully authentic or whole until all of life's experiences have been integrated into the personality, brought into full awareness, and released from the unconscious. There are therapists who specialize in voice therapy by addressing the subconscious mind represented by the body where the emotions are stored. My advice is to be cautious when beginning therapy, as the therapist must be of the highest quality and skill, and fully licensed. The danger present is to repeat the trauma and further anchor it in the psyche.

Crystal Singing Bowl Therapy

World cultures have recognized the importance of music and sound as healing tools for millennia. Ancient civilizations in India, China, Africa, Europe, and among indigenous peoples, such as the Australian Aborigines, the Maori of New Zealand, and Native Americas, have used sound to heal and achieve balance from within for thousands of years. The Tibetan Buddhists still use tingshas (bells), chimes, metal singing bowls, dharma horns, and chanting as the foundation of their spiritual practice.

In Bali, Indonesia, the trance-inducing gamelan (tuned metal instruments struck with mallets), gong, and drum are used in ceremonies to take listeners and musical performers into deep meditative states. The Australian Aborigines and Native American shamans use vocal toning and repetitive sound vibration with instruments created from nature in sacred ceremony to adjust any imbalance of the spirit, emotions or physical being. As you are aware, I have personally experienced the icaros of Shipibo shamans in sacred ceremony and the effect was life changing.

Recently, in the West, we have discovered that singing bowls, created from 99.99 percent pure quartz crystal, are powerful healing tools. Interestingly, the physical body has a natural affinity to this molecular shape as the human body is composed of many crystallite substances. Our bones and teeth are crystalline in their cellular structure, as is the liquid crystal-colloidal structure of the brain. Even on a molecular level, the biochemistry of the subcellular enzyme-containing structure, our cells contain silica, which balances and facilitates our electromagnetic energy flow. The human body is literally singing with frequencies and vibrations.

We know that chakras, bones, and organs in our bodies all possess different resonant frequencies—*resonant* meaning, the frequency at which they optimally vibrate. When an organ or part of the body is not in harmony or "vibrationally out of phase" with the rest of the body, that is a disease. A body is in a healthy state of being when each organ is in harmony (resonance) with the entire body organism.

We can assess a harmonious state by observing the balance within the chakra system (either by visual assessment, kinesthetic assessment, or by utilizing a pendulum). If an imbalance is found, using the sounds of crystal bowls a sound therapist can break up, dissolve, and release blockages that initially began in the light or etheric body. These imbalances can be caused by negative thoughts, toxic environment, unhealthy diet, fear, anxiety, worry, or stress, to name a few causative factors.

By aligning to the signature waveform of the crystal singing bowl, the body begins to express a more harmonious condition. This is because the sound transmits a pure holographic template of light that corresponds to the octaves of sound present within our etheric bodies. Since sound frequency can be translated into color frequency, the body may be seen as a color wash of visible frequency that produces an auric color field which can reflect all of the emotional states of consciousness.

To further explore this, I refer you to Kirlian photography. We may now assume that the visual spectrum has correlating wave frequencies in the auditory sound spectrum. There are seven musical notes that correspond to the seven colors of the rainbow, and these are also related to the seven main chakras, which in turn correspond to different glands in the endocrine system. The pure tone of crystal bowls produces a vibrational sound field that resonates the light body and chakras as well as the corresponding physical area; thus, it creates a "retuning" of the receiver back into a heightened level of etheric radiance, clarity, and physical wellbeing.

Note that while the etheric body may be tuned by the sound it takes time for the physical body to respond to the newly created landscape. Barbara Brennan, Ph.D., D.Th., a well-known leader in the field of energy healing and author of the seminal book *Hands of Light,* told me after a private session with her that the physical body responds to the energetic change in the etheric body in approximately six weeks. Although I only saw Dr. Brennan once, the single session I had with her was powerfully effective. I cannot speak for other energy healers who might require multiple sessions to get similar results.

My appointment with her happened in the early 1980s. I had been experiencing severe lower abdomen pain for over six weeks and had not had relief from medication. I was desperate, as the pain was constant. I walked into her office and as I stood in front of her she immediately said, "You have recently been probed." I will never forget those words, as the week before I had undergone an exploratory procedure at a hospital where I was indeed probed.

Dr. Brennan put me on a treatment table, surrounded me with crystals, and began sounding above my body with her voice. At times her voice was quite loud and at other times she used crystal singing bowls to clear heavy energy. I physically could feel the energy in and around my body moving and I also had an emotional release as I remembered an incident of abuse that I had suffered as a young woman. She consequently told me that root of the present physical condition was this abuse and that she had dissolved the imprint of that incident and knit together the damage—a tear in my etheric body. In six weeks, I had no more pain.

Like a powerful radio transmitter, the crystal singing bowls transmit energy in the form of white light sound filling a person's aura (energetic body), and physical body with vibrational radiance. This radiance holds, within its holographic sound, all expressions of frequency and vibration: the seven main colors of the rainbow, the colors of each chakra, and the seven notes in a musical octave. As a result, there is a positive shift in consciousness and a profound expansion of awareness. We then grow closer to our original selves and begin to reflect this radiance in our physical form. We become physical and spiritual carriers of this radiant light, capable of healing and uplifting all.

A Chakra Primer

In simple terms, the chakras are energy exchange vortices that facilitate energy exchange between our bodies and the quantum field that surrounds and connects all things. They have been described as *wheels* in the Hindu and Buddhist traditions because they appear or may be sensed, by those who can perceive subtle energy, as whirling wheels when they spin.

The inception points where these nonphysical wheels meet the physical body are located along the spine and extend like cones to the front and back of the body. Each of the chakras is "feeding" specific internal organs and nerve bundles. Chakras are the energy exchangers between the physical body (or matter), and the subtle (or etheric) body. They assimilate, exchange and emit life energy as traducers of the subtler energy in the field.

We now know that everything is energy, and everything vibrates, so if a person is saturated in negative emotions, thoughts, or impulses, the physical body will suffer. Conversely, a person who is a positive thinker and full of compassion and gratitude is probably a balanced being. In simply language, we become what we think and feel. So, for a vital and joyous life, a balanced and vibrant chakra system is imperative.

Now, the question is, how is this achieved? A good way to start is through meditation, balanced living, and physical care, exercise, breathwork, voice work, eating healthy nutritious food, restful sleep, and most of all, and *Above all else*, by living in love in action and thought. The most profound influence on creating a balanced state of the chakras is holding and creating internal peace. This allows the body to self-correct, to heal, and to balance.

Although there are many ways to move into our divine connection through love and stillness, I have found that music coupled with meditation can be extremely effective. It is enough just to fall in the musical arms of peace and rest. Molecular biologist Bruce Lipton, Ph.D., in his book *The Biology of Belief,* wisely says, "When it comes to stress, the answer to the ever young and energetic Tina Turner's hit song, "What's Love Got to Do with It?" is: "Everything!"'So, I ask you to choose LOVE, which is the great healer and carries the highest frequency vibration. Love all that comes into your experience, whether that is a person, experience, situation, idea, or observation. When your entire life is seen through the eyes of *love,* your chakras will balance.

Let questions of "Why did this or that happened to me?" become "What is my lesson here and what am I to learn."

Let "How can I love this person who has harmed me?" become gratitude for the opportunity to practice unconditional love for all. Yes, it may be hard, but the result is peace and health and joy.

I wish you success as you journey back to yourself, your true nature, and your divine self. This experience that we all share, of being souls incarnated on this most glorious planet, is beyond bliss. I invite you to be fully awake in this mystery.

Each chakra has distinct virtues and possibilities encoded in its energetic spin. The chakras are intrinsically linked to thoughts and emotions, so to lessen the impact of this aspect will not allow full healing. Oils, stones, foods, colors, and yoga poses all play an important part in balanced energetic flow, but the most powerful path to wholeness is the path of our thoughts (which come from our beliefs) and the energy of love.

Each of us has different ways of allowing love energy to flow through us. Some people listen to glorious music, some work with animals, some plant flowers and touch the soil of Mother Earth, some hike into the majesty of nature, some meditate in the spiritual cathedrals of the mind, some teach our children, some nurse the sick, and some conduct every second of their lives in the flow of love, seeing the divine in all things and people. So, do not discount any path if it seems to feed your heart and feels right. You are never out of the arms of love. Never. Just turn and accept the gift.

Let us now review specific ways to nurture each chakra.

Nurturing Your Eight Principal Chakras

We know that chakras are energy portals that take energy from the environment and help us to utilize it in a way that feeds our physical, emotional, and spiritual bodies. When the chakras function well, you experience health, joy, love, peace, wisdom, and connection with your divine expression. One way to nurture your chakras and self is to listen to the tracks on *Icaros: Chakra Soundscapes,* or another similar audio program, as each track is tuned to the resonant pitch of one chakra. That pitch becomes a foundation for the melodies which weave slowly within the triad built on that resonant pitch. As the musical triad is a chord of joy and resolution, it is easy to rest in those tonalities and experience peace.

The root chakra (*Muladhara*) is the chakra of stability, Mother Earth, and feelings of safety, trust, and security. Its color is red, and its resonant pitch is C. It is located at the base of the torso and governs the large intestine and pelvis. Essential oils which enliven the root chakra are clove, cedarwood, and rosemary. The mantra is LAM. Actions that develop the virtues of the root chakra are caring for animals, to create an environment of safety for them; exploring new hobbies, to broaden self-trust; and doing activities that have some anxiety around them, to break through the fear.

The sacral chakra (*Swadhisthana*) is the chakra of sexuality, vitality, and creative expression. Its color is orange, and its resonant pitch is D. It is located two inches below the navel and governs the sexual organs, kidneys, and bladder.

Essential oils which enliven the sacral chakra are sandalwood and myrrh. The mantra is VAM. Actions which develop the virtues of the sacral chakra are writing poetry, drawing, and painting, taking singing lessons, enrolling in a belly dancing class, and studying qigong or tai chi.

The solar plexus chakra (*Manipura*) is the chakra of will, sense of self, personal power, and self-control. Its color is yellow, and its resonant pitch is E. It is located two inches above the navel and governs digestion, the small intestines, and the autonomic nervous system. Essential oils which enliven the solar plexus chakra are lemon and chamomile. The mantra is RAM. Actions which develop the virtues of the solar plexus chakra are beginning a new project, taking public speaking classes, running a marathon, and volunteering as a tutor for children.

The heart chakra (*Anahata*) is the chakra of love, empathy, compassion, and generosity of spirit. Its color is green, and its resonant pitch is F. It is located in the center of the chest and governs the heart, lungs, and blood circulation. Essential oils which enliven the heart chakra are rose and jasmine. The mantra is YAM. Actions which develop the virtues of the heart chakra are volunteering at the local food bank, doing mission trips to locations in need of assistance, helping at an animal shelter, and adopting a stray animal. Being around animals is both a strong connection to earth energy as grounding and also the compassion of heart energy.

The high heart chakra (aka the thymic chakra) is the chakra of divine love for all creation and the connection with sacred geometry within the field of possibilities. It has no Sanskrit name that I am aware of. Its color is turquoise, and its resonant pitch is F-sharp. It is located between the throat chakra and the heart chakra. This chakra connects us to all sacred geometry within our natural world and is a portal to the cosmos. It has been called the "seat of intent." The pitches of F#, A#, and C# create a structure for consciousness to expand and connect with divine awareness. Essential oils which enliven the high heart chakra are frankincense, rose, and Idaho blue spruce. The mantra for the high heart chakra is OM. Actions which develop the virtues of the high heart chakra are total and complete trust that the universe is safe, knowing that all things happen for a reason, and we are the expression of love. Gratitude and compassion can then become the two guiding impulses that cradle us as we experience this mystery of indescribable beauty.

The throat chakra (*Vishuddha*) is the chakra of verbal expression in speaking the highest truth. Its color is blue, and its note is G. It is located at the larynx and governs the throat, esophagus, and trachea. Essential oils which enliven the throat chakra are eucalyptus and peppermint. The mantra is HAM. Actions which develop the virtues of the throat chakra are taking a public speaking course, teaching young people at your place of worship, or writing your life story with the wisdom gained.

The brow chakra (*Ajna*) is the chakra of intuition, perception, spiritual wisdom, and awareness. Its color is indigo, and its resonant pitch is A. It is located in the center of the forehead and known as the third eye. It governs the nervous system, eyes, ears, nose, and cerebellum. Essential oils which enliven the brow chakra are violet and lemongrass. The mantra is KSHAM. Actions which develop the virtues of the brow chakra are trusting your intuition, expecting synchronicities, and become relentlessly aware of everything around as you might see it in a dream.

The crown chakra (*Sahasrara*) is the chakra of enlightenment, self-realization, and connection with the divine. Its color is white and gold, and its resonant pitch is B. It is located at the top of the head and governs the brain as well as "feeding" energy to the entire organism. Essential oils which enliven the crown chakra are frankincense and rosewood. The mantra is OM. Actions which develop the virtues of the crown chakra are meditation, stillness in nature, quiet focus on beauty in nature, and listening to music.

Although this concludes our Chakra Primer, the following instruments are capable of activating and balancing the various chakras

Chakra Activating/Healing Instruments

Many instruments can be utilized for the purpose of sound healing. I have reviewed below the instruments that I have used in my sound healing practice. I suggest you go to a sound healing store that sells crystal singing bowls, Tibetan metal bowls, tingshas, and tuning forks and try them all. You will find the sounds that "feel right" to you. Remember, your body also is a resonating instrument. As a healer or sound maker, your clients and audience will entrain with your energy.

Tuning Forks

I was first introduced to tuning forks as vibrational therapy in France during the three-week Academy of Sound, Color, Movement, and Chi workshop I took with Fabian Maman. It is believed that tuning forks can interact with the universal life force energy that flows through the body by way of meridians and chakras. Energetic blocks caused by thoughts, trauma, environmental toxins, stress, anxiety, and exhaustion can interrupt this flow. Tuning forks create a vortex of sound and vibration that feeds into the physical and energetic body as a "reset" of pattern. Because they are tuned to specific frequencies, they can be very precise in interacting with the acupuncture points and meridian lines.

At the Academy, I was taught to use tuning forks tuned to the Pythagorean scale (aka the diatonic scale beginning with C). I used a full octave of eight tuning forks (C, D, E, F, G, A, B, C). Following the Hindu tradition of C being the root chakra, D the sacral chakra, and so on, as I described above in "A Chakra Primer," I could stimulate the vortex spin of the chakras that were out of balance. I found that when an acupuncture point was stimulated by the tuning fork, the corresponding meridian could be perceived by a tingling feeling. The theory is that when the correct tuning fork is placed (stem touching the body) the area, organ, or meridian will synchronize by way of entrainment to return to balance. Many sound practitioners are very adept at using tuning forks to return the body to a harmonic equilibrium.

Gongs

Gong baths have become popular means of energetic healing. If you have ever experienced this, you understand. The sound of the gong (especially if it is large) envelops your body with vibration that seems to penetrate every cell and crevice. It can be so intense that some people feel a bit faint with the power of the sound. I feel that it has the ability to break up disharmonious energetic patterns, much like the rattles that are used by South American shamans in their sacred ceremonies. Sometimes deep emotional issues, which are held in the body, are touched and released. Usually, there is an emotional component that accompanies this release, so I express a caveat here to approach this therapy with respect.

Tingsha Bells

Tingsha bells always come in pairs that are connected by a leather strap or chain. Like two small cymbals, these are used to begin and end meditation. They also have been used in aura cleansing and in the feng shui practice of clearing negative energy from a room or space. When struck together they produce a beautiful, clear tone, rich in overtones. The tingsha bells originated in Tibet and are called *Taa* in the Nepali language. It is believed that they were used in the shamanic ceremonies and rituals of the pre-Buddhism religion of Bon. The sound is beautiful in its simplicity and luminescence and can be used to begin and end group meditations. I use tingshas to complete a sound therapy session as the mind can focus and follow the very slow decay of the bell sound.

Sound Baths

A sound bath is part meditation and part listening. Typically, sound bath participants lie on the floor of a yoga studio or appropriate room and allow the sound vibrations to wash over them like warm waves of water. The instruments used in sound baths can vary depending on the purpose of the bath. However, crystal singing bowls, gongs, tingshas, tuning forks, slow shamanic drumming, and chanting can all be used to create the sonic experience. Sound bath enthusiasts report that they feel deeply calm and peaceful after a bath. Many times, participants fall asleep— and that's OK! The sonic waves are said to effect both the physical body and the energetic subtle body helping to alleviate depression, anxiety, and physical pain.

I would guess that there is also a release of serotonin, the feel-good neurochemical released during meditation. As a result, blood pressure drops, and the sound calms the mind. I recently enjoyed a sound bath at the Integatron, a dome-like structure near Joshua Tree, California. It was a lovely experience and was described as sound nutrition for the nervous system. I have facilitated sound baths as well, using just crystal singing bowls played in major triads with the fundamental tone matching the resonant frequency of each chakra.

One Vietnam vet who came to one of my sound baths using crystal singing bowls, Tibetan metal singing bowls, and tingshas, said it was the first time he had felt anything close to peace since he came home from war. He said it was like experiencing a space with no thoughts. I know it can be a very powerful practice for many people who experience it much like a sacred sound ceremony.

Chanting

Chanting is much like toning or therapeutic voicework in that the breath and vocal sound are involved, but it is vastly different in effect. Chanting is a rhythmical repetition (either silently or aloud) of a song, prayer, word, or sound. It is one of the most ancient spiritual practices and a part of most religions and spiritual paths. Chanting has been a part of ancient spiritual traditions probably from the roots of ritual devotion. We find *mantras* (a term drawn from a Sanskrit root meaning "quieting of the mind") used in chanting from all cultures and languages, including Hindi, Hebrew, Latin, English, and Arabic. Also, from African, Native American, Mesoamerican, Hawaiian, and certainly, the Indian cultures.

Christians commonly repeat AVE MARIA ("Hail Mary"), Jews recite BARUCH ATA ADONAI ("Blessed art thou, oh Lord"), Hindus repeat OM MANI PADME HUM ("Hail to the Jewel in the Lotus"), while Muslims repeat ALLAH ("God").

Other mantras include Sikh mantras, such as ECH ONG KAR SAT NAM SIRI WHA GURU ("The Supreme is one") and the Hindu mantra HARE KRISHNA, HARE RAMA ("Hail to Krishna and Rama").

Especially effective for me in my chanting practice is the classic kundalini yoga mantra RA MA DAA SAA SAA SAY SO HUNG. This mantra invokes the energy of the sun (RA), moon (MA), earth (DAA), and spirit (SAA) to bring deep healing and a merging with infinity (SAA SAY). SO HUNG translates loosely to "I am thou." I find that long after I have finished my chanting, the sound continues to cycle through my mind like a song that I can't get out of my head. The experience of chanting brings me great peace and a sense of profound calm. It opens my heart, stabilizes my breath, and gives my mind a focal point without the struggle to concentrate. What follows is an expansion of spirit.

The repetition of the mantra is a gift in its cycle of sameness. There is no goal, no ending, no expectation of activity, and no assumptions. There is no destination or need to rush to the end. The goal is flow. Simply to begin with OM or AUM is a splendid way to start to experience this island of peace. You will find that the humming vibration at the end is extremely pleasant as it can be felt stimulating the brow chakra and the crown chakra.

The breath taken into the soft belly is a way of opening the energy channels from the root chakra, through the heart and flowing through the crown. Additionally, chanting OM is associated with the experience of vibrational sensations around the ears, and it is thought that this sensation of vibration is transmitted through the auricular branch (ears) to the vagus nerve, promoting limbic deactivation. This simply means that the emotions of fear and anxiety are down regulated.

The vagus nerve is part of the parasympathetic nervous system that is in charge of returning the body to relaxation after stress or challenge. In Latin, *vagus* means "wanderer" in that this nerve wanders throughout the body connecting important organs. It reaches the brain, gut, heart, liver, pancreas, kidney, lungs, larynx, ears, and tongue. It is no wonder that stress (the opposite of relaxation) can cause colitis, upset stomach, hoarseness, high blood pressure, anorexia, and other digestive problems. When we have these symptoms, clearly the vagus nerve is not on line.

Chanting is more like vibrating than singing or toning, as it soothes at a cellular level and returns the spirit to oneness. I prefer to sit with my spine straight during my chanting so that the energy from my root chakra can flow easily up my spine. The deep breath is what begins this most mystical pump, this super-circuit.

When the breath is paired with calm, flowing sound, the parasympathetic nervous system responds, and all is translated into peace, healing, and deep harmony.

In his book *Becoming Supernatural,* Dr. Dispenza teaches that our personality causes our personal reality. Our thoughts, actions, and feelings drive the relentless machine that creates our lives and level of wellness. To change our reality, we must change either our thoughts, which drive our actions, our actions, which drive our feelings, or our feelings, which drive our thoughts. As you can see, it is an unending loop.

Chanting is a way to intercept and change feelings, thoughts, and actions, as the body, mind, and spirit are elevated to an evolved expression. We have seen that the vagus nerve, which is stimulated by chanting, can bring relaxed and peaceful feelings. With the peace come calm and loving thoughts and actions.

Meeting Tammy McCrary

In November 2016, while working as a sound therapist at the Integrative Healing Institute in San Antonio, Texas, I received a call from a woman who asked me if I could come to the intensive care unit (ICU) at St. Luke's Baptist Hospital to play crystal singing bowls for her brother who had just suffered a stroke. I immediately said yes, knowing that the sound of the bowls has a healing effect that can reduce high blood pressure by influencing the parasympathetic nervous system to return an anxious person to a state of calm. I imagined that this man would benefit from anything that would help calm him. Hospitals, although amazing centers of healing, can be places of anxiety and uncertainty. I ended up visiting the hospital three times and each time I went with my bowls the blood-pressure monitor in the hospital room reflected the calming effect of the sound of the bowls. That was very encouraging.

I was delighted to meet the family of this amazing man and learned that Tammy McCrary, his sister, was the woman who had reached out to me initially. I immediately liked her as we had so much in common: We shared a love of music and a passion for educating people about the power of music and sound. A close friendship and partnership evolved from these initial encounters and I now consider her a sister and colleague in manifesting a powerful vision of transformation through music and sound.

Tammy has a unique and rare background in the music business. She is a visionary, manager, director, author, and producer. Her story and profound insight into the music industry is inspirational and timely as we move into the twenty-first century.

Now, let's hear from Tammy.

EIGHT

....

EMERGING VISIONS OF SOUND HEALING IN THE TWENTY-FIRST CENTURY

In 2016, when I heard the news that my older brother, Mark, had been hospitalized after having a stroke, I really wanted to do something to support him. Everyone in the family was worried. Mark was semiconscious, and his status was very much touch and go. My sister Yvonne immediately flew to San Antonio, Texas, to be by his side. Though I couldn't travel at that time, having to care for my two sons, I still wanted to be able to support in some way. I knew the hospital was doing what traditional allopathic medicine does, but being a firm believer in holistic healthcare, with my whole heart I felt that we needed to supplement his treatment with care that was natural and healing.

A year earlier, I had hosted a retreat with my brother and two sisters. I wanted to introduce them to alternative healing modalities they could implement in their daily lives. We did acupuncture, reiki, and yoga, took amino acid supplements, and were "bathed" in the sounds of crystal singing bowls. Because my siblings are all musicians, the bowls resonated strongly with them.

Crystal singing bowls and Tibetan metal singing bowls may be used as a healing modality. Alternative medical practitioners create sound baths with instruments like these to assist the body in regeneration. Bowls are designed to produce vibrations of a certain frequency, or pitch, such as an F or a D, and are either held in one hand (if they have a stem) or set on a rubber ring. Then they are "sung" by gently sliding a rubber or suede mallet along the outer rim of the bowls.

Like my siblings, this was my first sound bath experience, so I didn't know what to expect. We lay down on the floor and relaxed as a sound healer played the bowls for us. As the sound of the bowls, which is as haunting as a human voice, washed over us, I found it calming and meditative. My mind relaxed and I gained a lot of clarity. I wasn't the only one who felt awed by the experience; each of us felt a similarly powerful feeling as the crystal singing bowls played. My sisters reported that the aches and pains in their bodies had disappeared, although it was also clear that the experience was different for each of us.

My brother was among those who were profoundly touched by the sonic experience at that retreat. Which is why I strongly believed that having crystal singing bowls played for him in the hospital would help him heal more quickly following his stroke. That was it! Once I had the idea, I only needed to find a sound healer in the locale of the hospital who could bathe Mark in the healing frequencies of the crystal singing bowls.

When I searched online for sound healers in the San Antonio area where my brother was hospitalized, the Integrative Healing Institute came up. I called and asked if they could have someone visit my brother and they connected me with Flicka Rahn. We spoke over the phone and immediately hit it off. Without hesitating, she said she would go to him the very next day.

Flicka took her crystal singing bowls to the hospital and set up in my brother's room. Yvonne was present and reported that they had never seen anything like that in the hospital. During the treatment, many others in the intensive care unit—doctors, nurses, and other patients—felt healing power emanating from those crystal singing bowls and asked what was going on in my brother's room.

My brother had an additional one or two sessions with Flicka over the next couple of days before my sister Yvette and I were able to join him and our sister Yvonne. When we got there, we surrounded him with love. We were all playing bowls around his bed at intervals and massaging his feet. We also made sure that he was getting healthy nutrition by convincing the doctor to allow us to add spirulina and chlorella greens to the nutritional supplement he was being fed through a feeding tube.

The effect of the nutrition and the sound-healing treatments on my brother were immediate; his blood pressure improved without medication. Even with the "trach" in his throat, which prevented him from speaking, he became more aware and communicative. In fact, Mark recovered so quickly that what was originally predicted to be months of recovery before he could leave the hospital, turned out to be a mere few weeks. He was soon able to get on a plane and come home to Los Angeles. We certainly didn't see that coming but were so happy that he was able to heal so quickly.

After my brother's experience with the crystal singing bowls, I was definitely a firm believer in using sound and music to heal. That sound healing was powerful and profound shouldn't have been a surprise to me. I grew up in Chicago in a musically talented family and have been uplifted and surrounded by music all my life. Some of my favorite memories are of me and my cousins organizing concerts in my Aunt Barbara's basement. I would sing a song or two but enjoyed being the facilitator and organizer. I was the only girl in the bunch of boy cousins my age, and I would corral them into playing air guitar on their tennis rackets, strumming along to songs like "Strawberry Letter 23" by the Brothers Johnson.

While my cousins and I were performing a "sold-out concert" to all eight of our family members in attendance, my eldest sister, Yvette (professionally known as Chaka Khan), was selling out shows to thousands all over the world. My second-oldest sister, Yvonne (professionally known as Taka Boom), was also enjoying a thriving career as a singer. Mark would later enjoy his own success a singer-songwriter. One of his hit songs, "Da Butt," which was featured in the 1988 Spike Lee film *School Daze*, still earns him significant royalties even today.

While I knew my family members were gifted, it was during college that I first became aware of the profound capacity that music has to heal. I worked with artists at the University of California, Berkeley, through SUPERB Productions, an organization that produced the concerts on campus. It was my job to be the artist liaison, including greeting them, preparing their dressing rooms, and making sure they were comfortable, all the way through to seeing them perform. A light bulb went off for me when I saw how the audience was emotionally impacted by the music. I thought that it was powerful, and I wanted to be involved in some way.

When I entered college, I originally thought that I wanted to become a business manager, but then I learned that this would involve sitting in an office, crunching numbers, and I decided I wanted to do more creative and collaborative work. Artist management was more interesting to me. I left school and began my career as an artist manager by developing the all-girl, multiracial singing group Pretty in Pink featuring my niece, Milini Khan, as the lead singer. The group had some wonderful successes, after which I went on to manage my former husband, Howard McCrary, and then my eldest sister, Chaka Khan.

When I met with Flicka at my brother's bedside in San Antonio, it was the start of my deep dive into the many aspects of sound healing. We knew we wanted to work together to bring this powerful modality to more people. First, we did a workshop in Los Angeles with some artists that embodied much of what is shared in this book and was also entitled the Transformational Power of Sound and Music, which went very well. Then we were invited to do a workshop at Agape International Spiritual Center, and subsequently reached out to Eric Rankin and Alanna Luna, who were deeply involved in making the 2015 film *Sonic Geometry*. Through them I became more aware of the groundswell of artists who have raised their consciousness and are involved in the 432 Hz movement to restore optimal tuning in the music industry. The four of us were next joined by Debbie Littrell to create a group called the Transcendence Experience, whose mission is to create fully immersive, sensory experiences that I, for one, firmly believe are the next and best step in healing and interactive entertainment.

Imagine going to a concert not just to be entertained, but to be physically healed. If the artistic community consciously uses music and sound to heal, we can ignite a modern-day renaissance and initiate a global transformation. When you are in the music industry, as I was for twenty-five years as an artist manager, you get inundated with everyone frantically looking for the next big thing, whether that is the next big sound, the next big trend, or what have you. I firmly believe that the next evolution in music is something much deeper: a reemergence of the ancient, healing sound frequencies integrated with contemporary music to elevate the soundtracks of our everyday lives.

The Reemergence of Music and Sound as a Sacred Healing Medium

"You know, I've been singing for forty years, but I can just look at the audience and I feel like they want more from me," Chaka once told me.

My sister relayed this observation to me a few years ago while we were having a conversation about the next project she would record. She didn't want to do another "love song CD," because she felt that the audience was yearning for more than just being entertained, that they really wanted to be fed on a deeper level. As destiny would have it, the opportunity was recently presented to do just that. My dear friend Mynoo Maryel of the World Dignity Forum introduced me to the Consul General of India, New York, who commissioned me to produce an audio and video recording of the classic Indian bhajan (devotional song) entitled "Vaishnava Jana To" in honor of Mahatma Gandhi in celebration of his 150th birthday (October 2nd, 2018) for a global campaign.

"Vaishnava Jana To" was a song that Gandhi would always sing prior to going into prayer. This song represents the principles that Gandhi so strongly stood for.

I was able to bring Chaka and one of India's most revered artists, Sonu Nigam, together for this momentous occasion to record this classic bhajan. Our collective intention in recording this song is to inspire a global remembrance of Mahatma Gandhi and the love, peace, and dignity that he so powerfully represented.

For all of my life, I've been aware of the healing power of music and its ability to elevate our moods and transform an environment. I can recall my parents having an argument when I was a small child and my mother putting on music after my dad had stormed out. Even then I was aware of music bringing joy back to my mother and restoring a sense of peace in our home.

As I grew older, as a teenager and young adult, I experienced how sound and music connects one to Spirit. I would attend Baptist church services and literally feel an energy rush through my body as I listened to and sang along with songs sung by the choir in a state of praise and worship. When I was baptized (for the second time) at sixteen, the pastor who baptized me insisted that I speak in tongues after the baptism to consummate it and assure him that I was then "filled with the Holy Spirit." My experience of speaking in tongues was very powerful and emotional. When I spoke in tongues, I just allowed the sound to flow from me without thinking about what was coming forth. What came forth filled me with overwhelming emotion.

Having had many different types of spiritual experiences, I could best describe it as a form of meditation. When you meditate, you release the thinking mind and allow yourself to connect with the Divine, universal consciousness, God, or whatever else you might choose to call that connection. Speaking in tongues could be likened to the toning that Flicka describes in Chapter 7. When we tone, we are essentially communing with the divine aspect of ourselves.

The use of music to elevate and positively impact health and wellbeing has a long tradition, perhaps thousands of years. Sadly, in our modern era, using music for spiritual and healing purposes has often been relegated to the realm of the esoteric, considered nonscientific and even somewhat "woo-woo." You had to run in certain spiritual, metaphysical, or alternative therapy circles to experience the healing and spiritually empowering effects of sound and music.

The good news is that sound healing is once again making its way into the mainstream, where more people from all walks of life can benefit from it. Do an online search of the phrase SOUND HEALING and you'll find numerous sound healing centers, associations, meetups, and job listings or certificate programs to become a practitioner in the field. For example, Jeffrey Thompson, founder of the Center for Neuroacoustic Research in California, has turned to electronic music as a healing mechanism after studying the effects of sound on the body for thirty years. His treatments include the use of a sound bed with speakers and a headset, which can be set to emit any frequency.

SVARAM, a center in South India, is dedicated to exploring the role of musical instruments in sound healing. No access to a metaphysical store or sound treatment center? No problem! You can order your own set of crystal singing bowls online, as well as watch a streaming video to learn how to use them. Sound healing is truly reaching the masses.

Scientific studies on the physical and psychological effects of sound on living beings is also gaining ground, though much of the research has revolved around hearing disorders and the effects different frequencies have on biological systems. In 1839, Heinrich Wilhelm Dove, a Prussian physicist and meteorologist (who, incidentally, also was interested in global climate studies), discovered that when pure tones of slightly different frequency are played in each ear, the brain perceives a new tone or "beat." He realized that this perception existed in the auditory system, particularly the part that processes stereo—or binaural—sound.[1]

Dove was ahead of his time. His discovery did not have any practical applications until more than a hundred years later, when biophysicist Gerald Oster published a seminal article about auditory beats in the brain in the October 1973 issue of *Scientific American*. Oster wasn't interested in healing with binaural beats, but he did see potential in using his discovery to learn more about human perception and to diagnose disease.[2]

It turns out that if you have problems hearing binaural beats, you might be at risk for developing Parkinson's disease a condition that my former husband is currently challenged with. I find this connection to be interesting, as he is a brilliant singer, songwriter, and musician. I remember he would have excruciating migraine headaches. Maybe there is a sound healing solution for him as well?

Psychoacoustics, the study of sound perception and audiology, is a well-established field. Other scientists, particularly neurologists and those studying the physics of sound, are also becoming more interested in sound as medicine. For example, there are more than twenty studies on brain entrainment (using binaural beats to sync the brain waves in both hemispheres) that show how the practice improves cognitive deficits, as well as helps alleviate stress, headaches, pain, premenstrual symptoms, and other conditions.

The wisdom of our ancestors is also being considered more seriously. In 2017, an Ig Nobel Prize was given to a pioneering psychoacoustic study of the didgeridoo, an ancient wind instrument originating with the Aboriginal people of Australia. The Ig Nobel Prizes are awarded to encourage research that might initially make you laugh, but warrants a second, more serious look. The study was first published in *The British Medical Journal* and it explored how the unique blowing technique used in playing the didgeridoo can help with health issues such as obstructive sleep apnea (OSA).[3]

Researchers note that traditional beliefs about the didgeridoo's health benefits deserve further investigation. Acoustic studies conducted on the instrument show that the instrument emits sound components in both the infrasonic and the ultrasonic ranges, which are known to have positive effects on biological systems.[4]

Another study, published in 2017 in the journal *NeuroQuantology*, looked at the possible healing effects of conch shell frequencies.[5]

I believe we are on the brink of understanding the science behind sound healing, but—while we wait for research to catch up with our collective wisdom—we should trust our own instincts and experiences because the world awaits healing.

With the rise of social media and the digital sphere, we have never been so connected, yet so alone. Self-reported rates of loneliness are rising, according to a Mental Health Foundation survey, while our ever-connected, always "on" way of working is causing us to feel unbalanced and unfulfilled.[6] The millennial generation, those between ages eighteen and thirty-four, report higher levels of stress than any other age group.[7]A recent survey of members of

Generation Z, those following the Millennials, said that they feel more loneliness than previous generations.[8]

Collectively, we as a people are in need of healing and transformation. We are living in extremely turbulent, yet transformative times. To many, it may seem as though the world is coming to an end, and it is. Old models have died, and new ones are emerging to replace them. To a great extent, technology is driving this shift as we have evolved significantly in this area. Now we are being called to evolve our collective consciousness, so that we can help alleviate the pain of birthing a new world. We need to resonate with a higher, more divine frequency.

All signs point to a large number of us, particularly the younger generations, stepping up our healing game. Those same Millennials, when polled, are into meditation, exercise, massage, and healthy eating. They are driving up sales of new age music and are famously eschewing bar crawls for juice crawls. The youngest generations also reject materialism (and even capitalism) in great numbers, preferring experiences to stuff.

What sorts of experiences do they prefer? Music festivals are high on their lists: Eventbrite research reported in August 2017 that 29 percent of Millennials attended a music festival in the prior year, compared with only 17 percent in 2014.[9]Another survey found that 80 percent of Millennials are more likely to attend a festival or show featuring artists who are committed to positive change, while 81 percent want to be part of a likeminded community.[10]

It should be no surprise that the festival scene is shifting from getting wasted to embracing wellness, according to trend reports from Spafinder and other industry watchers.[11]For example, Festival No 6 in the United Kingdom featured Tibetan singing bowl sessions, didgeridoo healing, and gong baths.

It's clear that people are trying to tap into something more, to obtain a more meaningful healing experience in their lives. If our intention is to create a world and society with individuals who are about love and joy and peace, then we as music creators and consumers need to proceed with clear intentions and mindfulness.

Lucky for us, a few musicians are already showing us the way.

Sound Healing in Popular Culture

In October 2014, social media went wild because Prince joined Facebook. He marked the occasion by agreeing to participate in a three-hour Facebook Q&A with fans. He also famously waited until the entire three hours had passed before he decided to answer just one question.

It was from Emanuel Hymnes, also known as Dee J FoGee, who asked him: "Please address the importance of ALL music being tuned to 432 Hz sound frequencies???"[12]

I spent a significant amount of time with Prince in 1998 when my sister recorded her *Come 2 My House,* CD with him at his Paisley Park Studios in Minneapolis, Minnesota. He was truly an out-of-the-box thinker and very enlightened on many subjects, so I am not surprised that music's power to heal was on his mind in the last few years of his life. I love that this was the question that Prince answered, and his response was short but sweet: "The Gold Standard." He also included a link to an article, "Here's Why *You* Should Consider Converting Your Music to A=432 Hz," which was published on the Collective Evolution website in 2013.[13]

Prince is not the only artist who has been aware of the significance of the 432 Hz sound frequency; the number of performers who are recording in this frequency is growing. Artists rumored to have recorded in these frequencies include the Beatles and Michael Jackson, which could be one reason their music was so resonant.

I am heartened that so many artists in such a wide variety of musical genres are exploring this frequency. For example, Don Lotti of Dangermuffin (a rock band whose members subscribe to a holistic, plant-based lifestyle), recorded much of its fifth album, *Songs for the Universe,* in 432 Hz. Lotti has expressed his concern that the 440 Hz frequency that so many musicians record in sacrifices the music's potential and notes that Dangermuffin uses frequencies that achieve healing. "In the record, you can hear pitch shifts where we work with sound healing and frequencies that are harmonious with the human body," he said.[14]

There is still a lot that science has not explored in this domain, but, as Flicka noted in Chapter 5, tuning instruments to A432 does create a more "exquisite sound," compared to tuning done at A440. Many claim that the 432 Hz frequency is a mathematically more pleasing frequency, while a few have observed that this frequency borders on the divine. In the article Prince referenced on the Collective Evolution website, author Elina St-Onge writes: "It is said that 432 Hz vibrates with the universe's golden mean, Phi, and unifies the properties of light, time, space, matter, gravity, and magnetism with biology, the DNA code, and consciousness."[15]

You don't need to dig very deeply to find some examples to listen to: YouTube is rife with examples of music either originally tuned to 432 Hz or adjusted to do so. That said, it's difficult to find definitive proof that certain rock legends, including Bob Marley and Jimi Hendrix, actually subscribed to the 432 Hz philosophy. A number of audiophiles and engineers have speculated that these artists keep getting thrown into the 432 Hz mix because, in the age of recording on tapes, pitches on recordings could change as the tape stretched. I prefer to keep an open mind in these matters, because science continues to catch up with ancient wisdom.

When we try to get a sense of how deeply the concepts and practices of sound healing have permeated popular culture, we need to look even further than the 432 Hz club. As musicians spend more time honing their art, many of them report a deepening relationship to spirituality in their music and awareness of the healing aspect of performing.

For example, the Grammy Award-winning singer and songwriter India Arie released four record albums whose sales reached ten million around the world, but she abruptly walked away from the industry in 2009 because she had felt stifled in a role that did not feel authentic to her. She returned in 2013 with the release of a new album, *SongVersation*, which contained a strong spiritual element and she is profoundly aware of the power of music to impact the body.

"I think our subtle body—the eternal part of us that extends beyond our physical body—is effected by the vibration of sound. Sound actually moves the subtle body— it shakes it. Sound can make that subtle body grow or shrink or heal," she said in an interview with *Unity Magazine* in 2014. "To me, that's what prayer is, too. Prayer is a sound; it's an incantation. In my opinion, music at its best is prayer. And when there are lyrics, the words affect thought patterns and consciousness."[16]

Beck is another artist who has become intrigued with exploring the healing aspects of music. He wanted his most recent album, *Colors*, to be joyful. "I wanted the record to be [one of] those albums you put on, or you're in the car, and it just sort of elevates the mood a little bit—you just sort of feel better." he said in an interview with NPR for "All Sounds Considered."[17] He noted that this exploration was something he had to dig into, but that he knew from the outlook that he wanted the album to be filled with light.

Beck expressed his admiration of artists who bring an "intangible quality that makes you feel better" to their music. He tried to create this himself by writing from a place where he'd suffered but was also aware of the "very simple things that make you glad to be alive." Music, he added, provides solace and connection. "It can have a healing effect. So it's been a powerful force in my life."[18]

An increasing number of classically trained musicians are also tapping into the healing power of sound. Take Ivan Yanakiev, who told *Vice Magazine* that the first time he had heard an instrument tuned to 432 Hz (his friend playing Bach's "Cello Suite No. 1 in G Major" on his cello), it was as though God had spoken. "It was a channeling of pure light and love that vibrated through the whole room," he said. "It was new. It was brilliant."[19] In 2013, he formed the 432 Orchestra with another cellist, Alexandros Geralis. The group won "debut of the year" in 2015 for its explorations in the 432 Hz frequency.

Another classically trained musician is Helane Anderson, a soprano who has turned sound healer. In 2015, she released *Elemental Alchemy,* an album that introduces violinist Ben Powell. She and composer Anna Drubich also collaborated on a piece that features singing bowls with various instruments and a chamber orchestra. She explained that while classical music exists in a tonal system, sound healing is microtonal, which is incorporated in the instruments of Eastern religions. "The sound itself accesses parts of the brain and produces alpha, delta and theta waves, which are the brain waves associated with high-level meditation. The sound, in a way, allows the brain to shut off, which is something we have a great deal of trouble with in our modern-day lives."[20]

As I look at all the examples of sound healing in popular culture, I am certain that there is a burgeoning awareness, a growing consciousness that is calling us to heal. I think music has such a huge part to play, not only in personal healing, but in healing ourselves as people, because it is such a powerful medium, bridging culture and class. It speaks to everybody, regardless of language. Music is also a place where you can deliver messages and teachings around so many issues that need to be addressed in our world. As artists are being called to help bring about change on this planet, the question remains as to how they can best take on this responsibility.

The Responsibility of Music Creators

When we talk about the potential that music and sound have to heal us, we must address the energetic connection that musicians have with their audiences. I have been professionally involved in the music industry since I was a teen, so I have seen and felt this energetic connection for myself countless times. It is simply glorious when the audience connects with the music and is uplifted by it.

I am also excited about all the healing potential of music, especially given my recent experiences with the healing of my brother following his stroke and my own work with Flicka. As has been touched on throughout this book, music, by its very nature, transcends the boundaries of language, class, and culture. Ancient cultures knew and tapped into this wisdom. Indigenous cultures have often been better keepers of traditions of healing with music than modern ones.

Don't misunderstand me: I love the entertainment aspect of music, because it can be a force for good. I simply believe we also have a sacred responsibility, as music creators, to be conscious of its healing power and to use our gifts to heal others. Oftentimes artists will say: "I am not responsible for what people think or feel. I'm just creating." But when you are on a stage or appearing on any performance platform, not necessarily as a huge artist, but *especially* as a huge artist, you are delivering something, putting something out there, and with that comes a level of responsibility to your audience.

If you've come this far in the book, you understand the visceral and emotional impact that the energy of music has on the body, mind, and spirit. Studies show how music vibrationally affects people's spirits and physiology. Understanding the nature of energy, frequency, and vibration is important because once you grasp the distinctions between various manifestations of energy you can consciously direct the energy you produce to ensure it benefits others.

It is unfortunate that the music industry itself often functions in a way that is detrimental to this powerful, creative healing connection and experience. Musicians—especially those who are reaching massive audiences or are on the cusp of breaking out in their careers—never operate as sole creators. They share creative control with others, tending to amass a team of writers, producers, managers, and marketing people, all of whom have a stake in the artist's career. Whether we like it or not, professional musicians are pressured to gauge their success on how marketable their music is and if it is riding a particular social wave. Artists feel a need to continue to earn more and more money. As a result, they will likely find themselves creating music at one time or another that does not reflect their own authentic style of expression. It is easy to end up creating from the wrong intention or objective once you have been swept up in the momentum of the music industry.

When the business side of music is overemphasized, it creates a rigid structure that has kept many artists from realizing their highest calling. In the realm of art-as-entertainment, where profit is the primary motivation, there isn't a lot of thought or attention given, ultimately, to how the end receivers are going to respond to the music. How does the music make them feel? What kind of energy is being sent out and is it raising the vibration of the audience?

I recall when Chaka was recording her tenth and final album for Warner Brothers Records. She was assigned an A&R person who suggested that she emulate another artist (whose name I shall not mention) who, ironically, had grown up listening to Chaka's music and even covering her songs. An A&R or "artists and repertoire person" is responsible for helping the artist identify songs and producers for a project. Essentially, Chaka was being asked to compromise her genuine expression to create something that the A&R person felt would have more marketability. In the end, Chaka severed her relationship with Warner Brothers because she was being asked to focus solely on marketability rather than on writing and recording songs that honored her own authentic voice and intent.

Experiencing this single-minded pressure to produce for profit can cost a performer bits of their soul, particularly if that performer is young and just starting out in the industry. I was particularly moved by an interview that Alanis Morissette gave to Oprah Winfrey a couple of years ago. As you may recall, Alanis rocketed to fame at the age of twenty-one with the release of her third album, *Jagged Little Pill*, but her success came at a steep price. Her songs for that album came from a deeply personal space and she went from playing small venues to huge concert venues practically overnight. She told Oprah that she did not really know who she was at that time and she had mistakenly thought that fame itself would be a balm for her pain. Under extreme pressure to present a superstar persona to the public, she found that she felt more isolated than ever, rather than experiencing the connection she longed for.[21]

It has taken Alanis a long road to find healing and she reports that her struggle with pain is ongoing, but she seems to be at a new place of self-acceptance and self-awareness. "One of the big lessons I have learned over the last little while, if I could become comfortable with pain, then there won't be living in the future all the time, that one day, if I will be happy," she told Oprah.[22]

India Arie has also observed how the music industry can unmoor artists. "I can't count how many times I have seen young people come into the business, and then their natural inclination shifts to accommodate what is more commercial. Their energy and all that magic they had is gone. It happens *all the time*," she told *Unity Magazine*.[23]

I can think of numerous examples of artists who are distracted from their purpose, who realize that the millions they make and the rewards, at the end of the day, do not necessarily make them fulfilled and happy. Ultimately, we all want to be able to affect other people in a way that elevates their lives. It's our God-given purpose.

So, what is an artist to do?

I have been pondering this question a lot, particularly through my work with Artistology, the academy I founded to help artists achieve at the most profound level. I developed the Artistology Method (TAM) to empower artists. The Artistology Method is an effective strategy for being able to work with intention and healing in your performance career.

The Artistology Method is particularly important because the music industry is experiencing a time of upheaval and rapid change. Like many other industries, the internet has significantly disrupted the music industry, and the upside of it is that artists can create a direct relationship with their audiences. Now an artist has more choices than ever to take control of his or her destiny. There are seven billion-plus people on this planet who can resonate with your unique experience and artistic expression. If you consciously practice expressing at a higher vibrational state, you'll always be fulfilled as an artist.

Artists are the architects of our future. There is a direct correlation between the messages that are delivered through music, film, and television, and even gaming and the society that is manifested. If we want to see a saner and more peaceful world, artists must take responsibility and lead.

The first question an artist must ask is this: What is the message I am here to deliver? I teach a whole course around this, but in a nutshell, you can use the hero's journey as a structure to discover what your journey has been, what your life has taught you, and what you are in turn here to teach and share with others.

When an artist wants to tap into the power of music to heal others, it's vital to go on this journey of self-awareness and healing. The energy you share in your performance is a direct reflection of your own state. One of the core strategies I think are important is really tuning into yourself, and the quickest way to do that it is through meditation, prayer, or a similar methodology. What you are doing is connecting with the divine aspect of your true self.

Flicka and I, in partnership with Daniel Wyman and Alanna Luna, have created a mobile app called Innergy Tuner that helps a person "tune in and tune up" their emotional state by listening to sonic prescriptions of music created in 432 Hz by Flicka and her music partner, Daniel Wyman. To accompany the sonic prescriptions, Innergy Tuner also includes visuals created by Alanna Luna designed to balance each of the body chakras. The Innergy Tuner app is a tool that was designed to assist individuals in elevating their emotional or vibrational states and balancing their chakras.

There are also a number of guided meditations and visualizations you can find on the internet or in audiobook form, or you can find a place to practice near you. Experiment until you find a spiritual and meditative practice that helps ground you and keep you focused on your authentic expression. You will likely find that is something that will become a daily practice, an ongoing visit to a source of strength and knowingness that lives within you.

Don't be discouraged if it doesn't happen right away; it often takes time to peel back the layers of ego, the masks we wear to please other people, until we can find that voice inside us that has been waiting to step onto the stage all along.

Intentionality is also an important aspect of using your gift as a force for healing. I understand that everything is not sunshine and roses, and how you choose to express may not always be at a high vibration. Even if you are coming from a state of low energy, or a low vibration, the intentionality you set is vital. If your intention is to bring a listener and/or yourself into a better space through that expression, that purpose and energy will be conveyed through your performance space.

Finally, I encourage musicians to explore recording at a 432 Hz frequency. You can also convert your music from 440 Hz to 432 Hz using Audacity and other tools. If you search online, or consult with recording engineers, it is a simple process and one well worth undertaking. As you play in this frequency, make sure to be mindful of the responses of your listeners and please feel free to forward your experiences to us by visiting the website of The Transcendence Experience: Lifein432.com.

Now, more than ever, we need artists and arts supporters who understand the power of music to step forward and light the pathway to peace and healing for all.

AFTERWORD

··

"How can I help?" is a question that I have heard countless times as I speak to people who feel connected to music and sound as healing paths. I trust that after reading this book you have a more comprehensive view and understanding of how sound heals. To reveal the profound power of this ancient art, we have delved deeply into the healing aspects of sound and music.

I hope it is evident to you that you do not have to be a musician to be a sound healer. Sound healing can be as simple as feeling love and channeling that emotion into your voice as you greet another person. You can expand your resources for healing by purchasing a crystal singing bowl that anyone can learn to play. Listening to music that is calm and lyrical can immediately affect your emotional and physical state and those around you. I recommend that you try the therapeutic suggestions in this book and find the ones that you find effective and enjoyable. Your personal experience and the result of your own healing will be valuable information as you begin to offer the rich and varied therapies to others.

Tammy and I believe that music is the most effective bridge to experience an evolved consciousness. Our deepest wish for humanity is that all of us come to know that we are far more than the limited views we hold of our personalities. From the perspective of unity, joy, compassion, and gratitude, humanity will fully embrace the vision of peace in our time. We feel that sound healers are the alchemists of this emerging reality. As Tammy has pointed out, musicians are the architects of the future. Singers, chanters, musicians, lovers of music, meditators, dancers, artists, writers, and healers of all kinds can begin to join hands and take us toward that vision. We are *all* of these things. We are all one.

ACKNOWLEDGMENTS

Flicka Rahn:

My deepest thanks to Tammy McCrary, who inspired me to write this book. Her guidance, wise counsel, and inspiration were a constant support throughout this journey. Without her brilliant vision of our mission of healing through music, I would not have ventured into this experience. She is a true sister.

A special thanks to Stephanie Gunning, our editor, who guided me through the labyrinth of unknowns for a new author. She has been amazing, and I have deep respect for her honest direction and encouragement.

A huge part of the presentation of this book, Alanna Luna has contributed her genius and deep cosmic knowing in the preparation of the graphic art. I am profoundly grateful.

My overflowing gratitude and thanks to my husband, Paul, for his love, unfaltering faith in me, and unending support. The humor and lightheartedness of my daughter, Kristann, was a source of energy and constant support. You hold a huge part of my heart.

For her guidance and unconditional love, I thank Dr. Marge Barlow. With her guidance and encouragement, she mirrored back to me my potential and wholeness. I consider her my Obi-Wan Kenobi with a little Yoda mixed in for lightness.

A special thanks to my university colleagues Arlene Long, Brad Kisner, Dr. Kelly Quintanilla, Dr. Sam Logsdon, and Dr. Diana Sipes, as well as the Texas A&M University–Corpus Christi community that supported the courses I taught on music and sound healing.

To my parents, Henry and Evelyn Rahn, my profound gratitude for giving me countless piano and voice lessons, for encouraging me to follow a dream to be a musician, and for their constant and overflowing love for me.

My beloved brother, Russell, who would sit with me for hours dreaming up potential projects, music workshops, and adventures into the Amazon. Always a part of these dreams was his encouragement to "live big." I love you, brother.

My deep kinesthetic and spiritual understanding of the human voice began with my extraordinary teacher Hank Hammett. You are a master teacher and I am singing today because of your guidance. My deepest thanks.

To my colleague and friend Ruth Friedberg who guided me through the rich world of American art song as we sang and lectured our way across the world. Thank you for sharing your passion for music.

Tammy McCrary:

My most sincere gratitude to Flicka Rahn for her trust and willingness to allow for new possibilities to emerge. Her brilliance, compassion, and artistry inspire me daily and are what has inspired this book.

A special thanks to editor Lori DeBoer, who assisted me in drafting Chapter 8, and Stephanie Gunning, the book editor who helped Flicka and me bring the book to fruition. Their guidance and support have been true blessings.

I thank my family for their presence in my life: My mother for the gift of life and her unyielding support; my father for his transcendent love; my sister Yvette for being one of my greatest teachers; my sister Yvonne for being a shining example of reliability and responsibility; my brother, Mark, for being my daily dose of the perfect balance of intellect and humor; my son Tallon for showing me what it means to 'be in the now'; my son Tyler for his brilliance as an artist and openness to learning what is shared on these pages; and the rest of my amazing family for what each of them has contributed to our collective present.

I thank my best friend, Veronica, and her husband, LaRosa, for their loyal friendship. My daily talks with Veronica were a constant source of inspiration.

I thank Alanna, Arlene, Ayelet, Carrie, Charles, Chaz Daniel, David, Debbie, Dierdre, Eric, Erica, Gina, Gwen, Hanan, Jamie, Jeff, Jody, Keith, Laura, Marcina, Marjorie, Mike, Monique, Mynoo, Nia, Stacy, Steve, Tara, and the rest of my ever-expanding tribe of amazing friends that share my passion to inspire, empower, and heal others.

NOTES

Chapter 1: A World History of Spiritual Music That Heals

1. "Sound Therapy: Taking a Holistic Approach to Life," Brainwave Power Music (accessed September 1, 2018), https://www.brainwavepowermusic.com/home/blog/ sound-therapy-taking-a-holistic-approach-to-life.

2. Hermes Trismegistus. *Corpus Hermeticum*, translation by G.R.S. Mead (1906). This text was originally published by the Theosophical Publishing Society (London) as part of the larger work *Thrice Greatest Hermes: Studies in Hellenistic Theosophy and Gnosis, Volume 2*. All Mead's translations are available through the Gnostic Society Library: http://gnosis.org/library/grs-mead/TGH-v1/index.html.

3. John Stuart Reid. *Egyptian Sonics* (CymaScope), https://www.cymascope.com/shop/products/egyptian-sonics-pdf-download.

4. "It's All about Frequency," Good Health with D blog (accessed September 19, 2018), http://goodhealth withd.com/its-all-about-frequency.

5. "Dorian Mode," Wikipedia (accessed September 1, 2018), https://en.wikipedia.org/wiki/Dorian_mode.

6. "The Pythagorean Theory of Music and Color," Sacred Texts (accessed September 19, 2018), http://www.sacred-texts.com/eso/sta/sta19.htm.

7. Guy L. Beck. "The Magic of Hindu Music: Exploring the Religious, Historical and Social Forces That Shaped Hindu Music and Now Propel It into the Future," Hinduism Today (accessed September 1, 2018), https://www.hinduismtoday.com/modules/smartsection/item.php?itemid=1515.

8. Ibid.

9. Excerpt from Jeff Strong. *Drumming to Drive the Brain: One Man's Music and its Impact on ADD, Anxiety and Autism* (Santa Fe, N.S.: Strong Institute, 2015), http://jeffstrong.com/2015/05/drumming-to-drive-the-brain.

Chapter 2: Common Elements in Sacred Healing Music

1. Joe Kimiya. "Behavior: Alpha Wave of the Future," *Time* (July 19, 1971), http://content.time.com/time/magazine/article/0,9171,905369,00.html.

Chapter 3: Musical Elements of Healing Sound

1. Rollin McCraty, et al. "The Electricity of Touch: Detection and Measurement of Cardiac Energy Exchange Between People," HeartMath Institute (1998), https://www.

heartmath.org/assets/uploads/2015/01/electricity-of-touch.pdf.

2. Rollin McCraty. "The Energetic Heart," *Clinical Applications of Bioelectromagnetic Medicine*, edited by P. J. Rosch and M. S. Markov (New York: Marcel Dekker, 2004): pp. 541–62.

3. Rollin McCraty, et al. "Modulation of DNA Conformation by Heart-Focused Intention" (Boulder Creek, CA.: Institute of HeartMath, Publication 03-008, 2003), http://www.aipro.info/drive/File/224.pdf.

4. Ibid.

5. Ibid.

6. Ibid.

7. Glen Rein and Rollin McCraty. "Modulation of DNA by Coherent Heart Frequencies," Quantum Biology Research Labs and Institute of HeartMath (accessed September 19, 2018), https://www.laskow.net/uploads/5/7/6/4/57643809/modulation_of_dna.pdf.

8. Definition of *ritual*, Oxford Dictionaries, https://en.oxford dictionaries.com/definition/ritual.

Chapter 4: Psychoacoustic Elements in Healing Music and Sound

1. Beverly Rubik, et al. "Biofield Science and Healing: History, Terminology, and Concepts," *Global Advances in*

Health and Medicine, vol. 4, supplement (November 2015), pp. 8–14,doi: 10.7453/gahmj.2015.038.suppl.

2. David Muehsam, et al. "An Overview of Biofield Devices," *Global Advances in Health and Medicine,* vol. 4, supplements (November 2015), pp. 42–51. Full text can be read here: https://www.iumab.org/overview-biofield-devices.

3. Park YongKeun, et al. "Refractive Index Maps and Membrane Dynamics of Human Red Blood Cells Parasitized by Plasmodium falciparum," *Proceedings of the National Academy of Sciences of the United States of America,* vol. 105, no. 37 (September 16, 2008), pp. 13730–35, https://doi.org/10.1073/pnas.0806100105.

4. Ibid.

5. Fabien Maman. *The Role of Music in the Twenty-First Century* (Redondo Beach, CA.: Tama-Do Press, 1997), p. 30–1.

6. Ibid., p.78–89.

7. Ibid., p.49–65.

8. Melissa Dykes. "Cancer Cure Suppressed for 80 Years: They're Finally Admitting Royal Rife Was Right," Truth Stream Media (August 8, 2017), http://truthstreammedia.com/2017/08/08/cancer-cure-suppressed-80-years-theyre-finally-admitting-royal-rife-right.

9. Alberto Güijosa. "What Is String Theory?" Instituto de Ciencias Nucleares (accessed September 19, 2018), http://www.nuclecu.unam.mx/~alberto/physics/string.html.

10. "Wave–Particle Duality," Wikipedia (accessed September 19, 2018), https://en.wikipedia.org/wiki/Wave%E2%80%93 particle_duality.

11. "Davisson–Germer Experiment," Wikipedia (accessed September 19, 2018), https://en.wikipedia.org/wiki/ Davisson–Germer_experiment.

12. "Einstein and Energy Fields," LifeShield Laser (accessed September 19, 2018), http://www.lifeshieldlaser.com/ albert-einstein.

13. Nick Strobel. "Spacetime," Astronomy Notes (accessed September 19, 2018), http://www.astronomynotes.com/ relativity/s2.htm.

14. Course material. "Module 5," Unified Field Theory Course/Resonance Academy, https://academy.resonance. is. Also explained by Nassim Haramein in this video: https://www.youtube.com/watch?reload=9&v=Yp8W_Zw 9hZI.

15. Stephen Winick. "Kumbaya: History of an Old Song," Library of Congress (February 6, 2018), https://blogs.loc.gov/folklife/2018/02/kumbaya-history-of- an-old-song.

16. Heinrich Schenker. *Harmony,* translated by Elisabeth Mann Borgese (Chicago, IL.: University of Chicago Press, 1980), p. 138.

Chapter 5: The Energy of Frequency, Forms, and Biofields

1. Ernst Chladni. *Discoveries in the Theory of Sound* (originally published in German as *Entdeckungen über die Theorie des Klanges* in 1787). Visit Max Planck Institute for the History of Science, Library, to see plates of these images: http://echo.mpiwg-berlin.mpg.de/MPIWG:EKGK1SP1.

2. Hans Jenny. *Cymatics: A Study of Wave Phenomena and Vibration, volume 2* (Newmarket, N.H.: MACROmedia, 2001), p. 120. Revised edition: http://blog.lewissykes.info/wp-content/uploads/Jenny_Cymatics.pdf.

3. John 1:1. *The Holy Bible, King James Version.*

4. "Rig-Veda," *Myths and Legends of the World*, Encyclopedia.com (accessed September 6, 2018), https://www.encyclopedia.com/philosophy-and-religion/eastern-religions/hinduism/rig-veda.

5. Jenny, p. 214.

6. Hans Jenny. *Bringing Matter to Life with Sound*, Part 1. https://www.youtube.com/watch?v=05Io6lop3mk.

7. Stephen Skinner. *Sacred Geometry: Deciphering the Code* (New York: Sterling, 2006), pp. 38–9.

8. Gary Vey. "It Hertz So Bad: The 432 vs. 440 Controversy," Viewzone (accessed September 19, 2018), http://www.viewzone.com/432hertz.html.

9. "What Is 432 Hz Tuning?" Attuned Vibrations (accessed September 19, 2018), https://attunedvibrations.com/432hz.

10. Eric Rankin and Alanna Luna. *Sonic Geometry: The Language of Frequency and Form* (2015), https://www.sonic geometry.com.

11. Ibid.

12. Ibid.

13. Ibid.

14. Tony Phillips. "The Sounds of Interstellar Space," Science/NASA (November 1, 2013), https://science.nasa.gov/science-news/science-at-nasa/2013/01nov_ismsounds.

15. Marty. "Fractal Frequencies and the Brain," Martyan Chronicles (accessed September 19, 2018), http://the-martyan-chronicles.com/2018/05/29/fractal-frequencies-and-the-brain.

Chapter 6: Physical and Emotional Impact of Healing Sound and Music

1. "Heart Rate Variability," HeartMath Institute (October 27, 2014), https://www.heartmath.org/articles-of-the-heart/the-math-of-heartmath/heart-rate-variability.

2. Ibid.

3. Rollin McCraty. "Music Enhances the Effect of Positive Emotional States on Salivary IgA," *Stress Medicine*, vol. 12, no. 3 (July 1996), pp.167–75.

4. John Hagelin. "Effects of Meditation on Brain Coherence and Intelligence," MeditationPlex (accessed September 19, 2018), http://www.meditationplex.com/meditation-

benefits/effects-meditation-brain-coherence-intelligence. Also see: http://www.hagelin.org.

5. Ibid.

6. Ibid.

7. Ibid.

8. "Anxiety: The Problems of Fast Beta Waves as Related to Anxiety, Insomnia, and Obsessive-Compulsive Disorder," Nu-Brain International (accessed September 19. 2018), http://www.nu-brain.com/anxiety.asp.

9. Antoine Lutz, et al. "Long-term Meditators Self-induced High-amplitude Gamma Synchrony during Mental Practices," *Proceedings of the National Academy of Sciences of the United States,* vol. 101, no. 46 (November 16, 2004), pp. 16369–73, http://www.pnas.org/content/101/46/16369.

10. Ibid.

11. Personal experience using many types of music for meditation.

12. Katy Koontz. "Listening in with Joe Dispenza," *Unity Magazine* (January/February 2016), http://www.unity.org/sites/unity.org/files/files/2016_UnityMag_Jan_Feb-Dispenza.pdf.

13. Simon Young. "How to Increase Serotonin in the Human Brain Without Drugs," *Journal of Psychiatry and Neuroscience,* vol. 32, no. 6 (November 2007), https://www.ncbi.nlm.nih.gov/pmc/articles/PMC2077351.

14. J.L. Harte, et al. The Effects of Running and Meditation on the Beta-endorphin, Corticotropin-releasing

Hormones and Cortisol in Plasma and on Mood," *Biological Psychology*, vol. 40, no. 3 (June 1995), pp. 251–65, https://www.ncbi.nlm.nih.gov/pubmed/7669835.

15. C.C. Streeter, et al. "Effects of Yoga Versus Walking on Mood, Anxiety, and Brain GABA Levels: A Randomized Controlled MRS Study," *Journal of Alternative and Complementary Medicine*, vol. 16, no. 11 (November 2010), pp. 1145–52, https://www.ncbi.nlm.nih.gov/pubmed/20722471.

16. Harte, et al.

17. Tonya L. Jacobs, et al. "Self-reported Mindfulness and Cortisol During a Shamatha Meditation Retreat," *Health Psychology*, vol. 32, no. 10 (October 2013), pp. 1104–9, https://www.ncbi.nlm.nih.gov/pubmed/23527522. Also see: University of California, Davis. "Mindfulness from Meditation Associated with Lower Stress Hormone," Science Daily (March 28, 2013), www.sciencedaily.com/releases/2013/03/130328142313.htm.

18. Ibid.

Chapter 7: Implementing Sound as a Healing Agent

1. Bruce Lipton. *The Biology of Belief: Unleashing the Power of Consciousness, Matter and Miracles* (Santa Rosa, CA.: Elite Books, 2005), p.162.

Chapter 8: Emerging Visions of Sound Healing in the Twenty-First Century

1. Esther Inglis-Arkell. "How a Scientist's Least Important Discovery Became His Most Famous," *Gizmodo* (November 16, 2015), https://gizmodo.com/how-a-scientists-least-important-discovery-became-his-m-1742623371.

2. Gerald Oster. "Auditory Beats in the Brain." *Scientific American*, pp. 94–102. https://www.amadeux.net/sublimen/documenti/G.OsterAuditoryBeatsintheBrain.pdf.

3. Milo A. Puhan, et. al. "Didgeridoo Playing as Alternative Treatment for Obstructive Sleep Apnoea Syndrome: Randomised Controlled Trial," *British Medical Journal* (February 2, 2006), p. 332, https://doi.org/10.1136/bmj.38705.470590.55.

4. J. Shashi Kiran Reddy, "On Psychoacoustic Studies of Didgeridoo," *British Medical Journal* (December 20, 2017), https://www.bmj.com/content/332/7536/266/rr.

5. Y.V. Suseela and JSK Reddy. "A Note on Possible Healing Effects of Conch Shell Frequencies," *NeuroQuantology*, vol. 15, no. 3 (2017), pp. 193–6.

6. Jo Griffin, et al. "The Lonely Society." Mental Health Foundation, 2010.

7. "Stress in America." American Psychological Association.

8. Vivian Manning-Schaffel. "Americans Are Lonelier Than Ever—but 'Gen Z' May Be the Loneliest," NBC News (May 14, 2018), https://www.nbcnews.com/better/pop-

culture/americans-are-lonelier-ever-gen-z-may-be-loneliest-ncna873101.

1. "Three New States about Millennials' Taste in Live Music," Eventbrite (August 16, 2017), https://www.eventbrite.com/blog/millennials-trends-in-music-data-ds00.

2. Ibid.

3. "2016 Trends Report," SpaFinder Online, https://www.spafinder.com/blog/trends/2016-report/well-fests.

4. Joe Lynch. "Prince's Three-Hour Facebook Q&A Yields One Actual Reply," *Billboard* (October 14, 2014), https://www.billboard.com/articles/news/6266816/prince-facebook-qa-one-reply.

5. Elina St. Onge. "Here's Why You Should Consider Converting Your Music to A=432 Hz," Collective Evolution (December 21, 2013), https://www.collective-evolution.com/2013/12/21/heres-why-you-should-convert-your-music-to-432hz.

6. "Frontman Dan Lotti on the Science in Dangermuffin's New Alum," Holy City Sinner (November 4, 2014), http://www.holycitysinner.com/2014/11/04/frontman-dan-lotti-on-the-science-behind-dangermuffins-new-album.

7. St. Onge.

8. Katy Koontz. "Listening in with India Arie," *Unity Magazine* (November/December 2014), pp. 26–9.

9. Robin Hilton. "Beck on Healing Through Music, the Deep Art of Pop and His New Album, 'Colors,'" All Songs Considered/NPR (November 9, 2017), https://www.npr.org/ sections/allsongs/2017/11/09/562866716/beck-on-healing-through-music-the-deep-art-of-pop-and-his-new-album-colors.

10. Ibid.

11. Chris Hampton. "The 432Hz 'God' Note: Why Fringe Audiophiles Want to Topple Standard Tuning," NOISE Department, Vice (May 12, 2014), https://motherboard.vice.com/ en_us/article/xywy74/the-fringe-audiophiles-who-want-to-topple-standard-tuning.

12. Jim Farber. "The Art of Healing with Sound," San Francisco Classical Voice (September 9, 2015), https://www.sfcv.org/ article/the-art-of-healing-with-sound.

13. Oprah Winfrey. "Alanis Morrissette: Is Happiness Temporary? (Maybe That's Okay)" Oprah's Super Soul Conversations (August 23, 2017), https://www.youtube.com/watch?v=YHIozeiOtiE.

14. Ibid.

15. Koontz.

RECOMMENDED READING

Andrews, Ted. *Sacred Sounds: Transformation Through Music and Word* (Woodbury, MN.: Llewellyn Publications, 1992.

Beaulieu, John. *Human Tuning: Sound Healing with Tuning Forks* (High Falls, N.Y.: BioSonic Enterprises, 2010).

Brodie, Renee. *The Healing Tones of Crystal Bowls* (Barnaby, B.C.: Aroma Art, 2000).

Campbell, Don. *Music: Physician for Times to Come* (London, U.K.: Quest Books, 1991).

Dewhurst-Maddock, Olivea. *The Book of Sound Therapy: Heal Yourself with Music and Voice* (New York, N.Y.: Simon and Schuster, 1993).

Emoto, Masaru, *The Hidden Messages in Water* (Hillsboro, OR.: Beyond Words, 2004).

Gardner, Kay. *Sounding the Inner Landscape: Music as Medicine* (Shaftesbury, U.K.: Element Books, 1997).

Gass, Robert. *Chanting: Discovering Spirit in Song* (New York: Broadway Books, 1999).

Gaynor, Mitchell L. *The Healing Power of Sound: Recovery from Life-Threatening Illness Using Sound, Voice and Music* (Boston, MA.: Shambhala, 1999).

Goldman, Joshua and Alec W. Sims. *Sound Healing for Beginners: Using Vibration to Harmonize Your Health and Wellness* (Woodbury, MN.: Llewellyn, 2015).

Govinda, Kalashatra. *A Handbook of Chakra Healing: Spiritual Practice for Health, Harmony, and Inner Peace* (Old Saybrook, CT.: Konecky and Konecky, 2009).

Holtje, Dennis. *From Light to Sound: The Spiritual Progression* (Temecula, CA: Master Path, 2000).

Jenny, Hans. *Cymatics: A Study of Wave Phenomena and Vibration* (Eliot, ME.: MACROmedia, 2001).

Keyes, Laurel Elizabeth. *Toning: The Creative Power of the Voice* (Marina del Rey, CA.: DeVorss and Co., 1973).

Maman, Fabien. *Healing with Sound, Color and Movement: Nine Evolutionary Healing Techniques* (Redondo Beach, CA.: Tama-Do Press, 1997).

Maman, Fabien. *The Role of Music in the Twenty-First Century* (Redondo Beach, CA.: Tama-Do Press, 1997).

Maman, Fabien. *The Body as a Harp: Sound and Acupuncture* (Redondo Beach, CA.: Tama-Do Press, 1997).

Mendes, João and Ramiro Mendes. *Sound: The Fabric of Soul, Consciousness, Reality, and the Cosmos* (Cheyenne, WY.: Quantum World Enterprises, 2015).

RESOURCES

To contact Flicka Rahn or Tammy McCrary, and for additional information on sound healing, please visit one of our websites.

The Transformational Power of Sound and Music Website
PowerofSoundandMusic.com

The Life in 432 Website
Lifein432.com

Flicka Rahn's Icaros Website
TheIcaros.com
Download free gift of music for High Heart Chakra (F#).

Tammy McCrary's Artistology Website
Artistology.com

Innergy Tuner App (to elevate mood and balance the chakras)
InnergyTuner.com

For bookings, please contact:
bookings@powerofsoundandmusic.com

Additional Resources

Barbara Brennan School of Healing
BarbaraBrennan.com

The Center for Neuroacoustic Research
ScientificSounds.com

The HeartMath Institute
HeartMath.org

Integrative Healing Institute
Natural Reflexes.com

Resonance Science Foundation
Resonance.is

Sonic Geometry
SonicGeometry.com

Tama-Do: The Academy of Sound, Color and Movement
Tama-Do.com

Terra Nova Mastering (for 432 Hz. audio mastering)
TerraNovaMastering.com

INDEX

ABOUT TAMMY MCCRARY

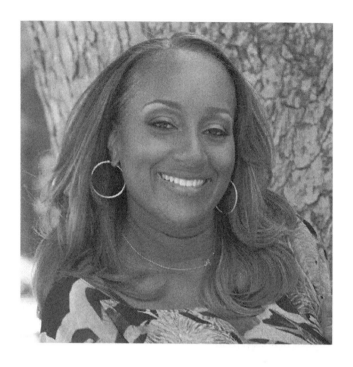

Tammy McCrary, CEO and chief inspiration officer of Artistology, is an entertainment consultant and entrepreneur. She has lived and breathed innovation and entertainment for more than twenty-five years. From her time as a hands-on artist manager and her role as a brand strategist to her success as a senior-level entertainment business executive and nonprofit sector leader, Tammy has excelled at reimagining what it means to be a music industry pioneer. A passionate proponent of collaboration, Tammy is a cofounder of the Transcendence Experience, a cocreator of the Innergy Tuner app, and coauthor of the best-selling book *Succeeding Through Doubt, Fear and Crisis.*

Tammy's visionary career began as a student at the University of California, Berkeley, where she worked as an artist relations coordinator with SUPERB Productions, the organization that oversaw the university's concerts. Eventually, that early experience with event production led to decades of professional work in artist management, as she successfully guided acts ranging from a pop girl group and an award-winning jazz singer and pianist to a legendary diva.

As a producer, Tammy's credentials are as varied as they are impressive. She executive produced the legendary Chaka Khan's *Funk This,* an album that garnered critical acclaim and two Grammy Awards, and she served as a producer of the 2013 Soul Train Music Awards. Tammy also coproduced and was featured in *Diagnosis,* a documentary about autism that won the Emerging Filmmaker Award at the Cannes Film Festival's American Pavilion showcase.

Driven by a desire to help those who are challenged like her son, Tallon, who has autism, Tammy cofounded two nonprofit organizations: The Chaka Khan Foundation and Colored My Mind. During her tenure as the chairman of the Chaka Khan Foundation, the organization raised $1.4 million in aid of autism awareness and research, while Colored My Mind was able to band together in 2011 with the National Black Caucus of State Legislators and National Hispanic Caucus of State Legislators to reauthorize the

Combating Autism Act of 2006. As a result of those joint lobbying efforts, the U.S. federal government committed to providing in excess of $3 billion for autism research and other services.

Following these diverse accomplishments, Tammy founded the Artistology Academy and Community to empower artists at every level of success. Whether they're just starting out, at the mid-level of their career, or enjoying great success in the music, film, or television businesses, through her experience, resources, and vision Tammy helps creative individuals take ownership of their artistic careers and utilize new technology in the most effective ways. Her mission is to inspire artists to collaborate and create products that make a positive impact in the world.

Tammy resides in Los Angeles, California.

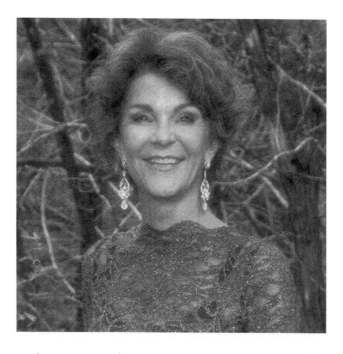

Flicka Rahn, M.M.Ed., M.Sc., is an internationally known vocalist, composer, and sound healer, with a distinguished career in academia teaching at a number of universities. A former associate professor of music at Texas A&M University, Corpus Christi, where she taught for twenty-two years, she has also served on the faculties of Brandeis University in Boston, Massachusetts, the Boston Conservatory of Music, and the University of the Incarnate Word in San Antonio, Texas. She earned a bachelor's degree from Washington University in St. Louis, Missouri, a master's degree in vocal performance from Texas State

University, and a master's degree in guidance and counseling from Texas A&M, Kingsville. Since 2015, Ms. Rahn has been practicing sound therapy at the Integrative Healing Institute in San Antonio. She is a cofounder of the Transcendence Experience and cocreator of the Innergy Tuner app.

As a vocalist, Ms. Rahn has sung major operatic roles throughout the United States. She has appeared as a guest artist with, among others, the Boston Lyric Opera, the New York Wagner Society, the Boston Concert Opera, the Minnesota Grand Opera, and the San Antonio Opera. She has graced the stages of major concert halls, including Carnegie Hall, Boston Symphony Hall, and the Boston Academy of Music. She had the distinction of having worked as a cantor for over thirty years at Temple Beth El in San Antonio. Her international recitals include appearances in La Paz, Bolivia; Toledo, Spain; and Puebla, Mexico, as part of a Cultural Music Exchange showcasing American art songs.

In 2012, as a Fulbright Scholar, she traveled to the Universidad Autonoma de Queretaro in Queretaro, Mexico, and taught courses on American art songs and American musical theater. She returned to Queretaro in 2015 to produce and direct musical presentations at the Proarte Escuela de Danza and the Centro Estudios de Musicales. In 2016, she continued her work in Mexico appearing with the Queretaro Symphony in their annual Opera Gala, performing solos and ensembles with Mexican vocal artists. She continues to have a large studio of classical vocal students in

Queretaro, Mexico. In 2017, she and Mexican tenor Andres Pichardo presented concerts in four cities throughout Mexico. In 2018, she returned to sing a concert in Mexico City with tenors Alberto Angel and Andres Pichardo.

As a composer, Ms Rahn's sacred and secular pieces for vocal soloists, choirs, and opera companies have been performed at universities, educational institutions, churches, museums, and temples. Her art songs are published in the series *Art Songs by American Women Composers*. In 2017, she and her musical partner, Daniel Wyman, recorded and released an album of meditation and healing music, *Icaros: Chakra Soundscapes,* which was inspired by her experiences of the improvised healing songs of the Shipibo shamans from the Amazon jungle in Peru.

In addition to her professional activity as a singer, composer, and teacher, Ms. Rahn offers sound healing therapy to clients at the Integrative Healing Institute in San Antonio, Texas.

Flicka Rahn currently resides on a horse farm in rural Texas. She is married and has a grown daughter.

Printed in Great Britain
by Amazon

42331914R00160